PARALLEL RECOVERY

A GUIDE FOR THOSE WHO LOVE SOMEONE WITH SUBSTANCE USE DISORDER

LISA KATONA SMITH, MED

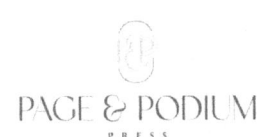
PAGE & PODIUM
PRESS

For Noah, Luke, and Tom, who gave me the reason and the room.
For the families who said yes to the journey.
For those still suffering, may you find the courage to love better.
And for the woman I used to be. You did it.

CONTENTS

INTRODUCTION

IF YOU LOVE someone who struggles with substance use disorder (SUD), your life has probably become difficult. In fact, it has probably sucked.

You don't understand their behavior, and you certainly don't support it, but every attempt to help them only seems to push them further away and makes *you* feel worse. You love your person deeply, and it hurts to watch their dangerous and unhealthy behaviors.

Whether your person is a parent, a child (regardless of age), a sibling, or a chosen family member, the reason this experience hurts so deeply is because you love them so much. You hurt *because* you love. That same love can provide an essential pathway to recovery, but the love you feel doesn't always translate to having influence over your person.

Parallel Recovery™ is a program that focuses on the foundation of connection to provide influence and mutual recovery from the harms caused by substance use disorder. Many programs focus on the individual with strategies to correct their behavior, get them into treatment, or otherwise "fix" the person with the disorder.

These programs are popular because they promise a solution, an end—they promise to make the pain stop. When you're worried about someone you love, sometimes all you can think about is making the pain stop.

The bad news is that there is no one-and-done solution. But there is a new way of living day-to-day that is focused on creating sustainability and connection as the foundation for achieving a life in recovery worth more than the life masked by addictive behaviors. Parallel Recovery invites families to do the active work needed to invite their loved one to join them on the journey to recovery. I call it "Parallel Recovery" because families need more than just support to get through these difficult circumstances. They also need an invitation and guidance in how they can move forward into a more sustainable future, becoming the model for recovery, developing new patterns of connecting and caring for themselves and their person, and ultimately, learning to love better.

The inclusive healing approach acknowledges that everyone in the family unit is connected and shares the burden of change. All of us can either play a role in the journey to wellness or we can participate in perpetuating the problem. Parallel Recovery empowers families with the tools needed to *choose* to work toward wellness, even when it feels impossible.

Today, the connection you have to your loved one may be strained, even fragile, but it can become resilient and honor each other's struggles and choices in those struggles. When that relationship is resilient, it can withstand the challenges of the journey to recovery. You can provide the strong and stable support system your person needs to recover from substance use disorder in the long term. But first, the entire family will need to do the hard work of reflecting, learning, communicating, and behaving in healthier ways with each other, sharing the burden of change and modeling a path to recovery for and with each other.

The commonly heard phrase "detach with love" suggests that in order to love your person and help them into recovery, you have to emotionally step out of the relationship. While stepping back can be a form of self-preservation, detachment is not love.

Parallel Recovery focuses on loving better.

You may not be able to help your person find their way back to stability and health—that is their job, and there are no guarantees in recovery—but emotionally checking out is not love. Love also isn't taking them by the hand and directing them to better choices. Nor is it attending all the meetings and reading all the articles, hoping you will uncover the perfect answer they haven't tried yet. You can't do the work of healing on their behalf. You can't "fix" them just because you want to so badly.

And that's okay. Because forcing someone to do what you want them to do because you are uncomfortable is not love.

Instead, you can come to the relationship with a spirit of curiosity and collaboration. You can step *into* the relationship with your person, the way they exist right now, and start the work of healing both your relationship and yourself. You can address your own needs and share the burden of change by inviting your person to work in parallel with you toward something better, more sustainable, healthier, and, ultimately, more loving for everyone. In doing so, you can help them find the connections they want to get better *for*.

With the right tools, you can nurture that connection without further participating in the harmful patterns that surround and propagate their substance use. You can maintain the relationship without letting the chaos upend your life or endanger your safety or wellness. The natural consequences of their behavior do not have to become your burden to bear to keep that relationship alive. Instead of focusing on detachment, control, and fear, you can focus on love and connection.

I understand what it's like to love someone who is struggling with substance use. It's painful and scary and isolating. I felt as though something had crept into my home and stolen my son. I had never expected it and was not prepared. We were not "those people." I was a teacher. We lived in a nice community. My son was a decorated soccer player, swimmer, and musician in the band.

For years, I searched for answers and help. Every day, he seemed to move further and further away from positive change. And from me. The traditional advice and models for support didn't help. It felt like the only message out there was that my son was choosing his path. As long as I allowed him to continue making that choice, I was keeping him in a cycle of addiction. If I tried to stop him, I was codependent. Those messages struck me as deeply flawed and incomplete.

The truth was that he was in pain. I was desperate to help him. Neither of us knew a different way.

Finally, I came to the realization that the changes I could control started with me. The starting point was to work on myself. To become the person I could be proud to show up as in this relationship, I had to love my son in a way that he could receive, separate from his behavior and as the person who had lost himself.

I wish I could say that realization alone changed everything. But it was only the beginning of a new way forward for me and my family that took, and continues to take, hard work, consistent intentionality, and mindfulness.

In the years since, I have helped hundreds of families find their own way forward, taking charge of their own recovery first in order to show up for and support the recovery of their struggling person. I have worked to shine a light on what I learned firsthand: Addiction is not just a disease that strikes individuals alone. Addiction is a family disease, which means recovery is for the whole family.

There is no wrong time to step into an intentional process of recovery with your loved one. Even if you've made mistakes in the past or tried things that didn't work—or even backfired—you can make a choice to try a different way forward. Choosing a new way can model for your loved one that change is possible.

But while there is no wrong time to begin the process, there is a wrong time to leave.

There are many insidious myths surrounding recovery from addiction. Many popular narratives describe a process of hitting rock bottom, getting into a spa-like treatment center for precisely twenty-eight days and nights, and "breaking the chains" of addiction for good through a regimented program of medical and psychological help.

If your family has been affected by substance use, you know that this seemingly simple progression is not the solution for most people. Even so, it can be difficult to let go of the idea that there will be, at some point, an end game. Families often hope that once their person seeks treatment, they will have achieved their goal; they can finally step away from the situation and leave things to the professionals. They can exhale. In reality, the moment your person seeks help is often the moment when your recovery is needed most.

The Parallel Recovery process is not about an individual getting treatment. It's about a whole family sharing the burden of change and entering a program of healing.

If and when your person completes a professional recovery program, you will be prepared to step up just as the professional treatment steps down. With Parallel Recovery, you will have the tools to continue open communication and support for the months and years after your person's engagement in recovery.

*

Not so long ago, my family spent Thanksgiving together in our home for the first time in years. Both of my kids were here, and both were healthy. Over the course of years, my son has built a meaningful life in recovery that allows him to thrive on his own terms. It was not a straight line. He has had professional help and our support, but the life he has now is one he built for himself. That life is sustainable for him, and it allows us to maintain our valuable connection and honest love for each other.

For many years, a traditional holiday was simply not an option for us, at least not in the way most people imagine it. Some holidays, we visited our son where he was living and spent time together there. Others, all we could do was meet him where he was existing—his head just above water—to offer a plate of food and a hug.

It was wonderful to have this holiday together, and I know many families would see this as an unqualified victory—the sort of success they dream of.

But those other holidays were also wins. Our yardstick, so to speak, for measuring that success was different because what was possible at each moment for each of us was different. We weren't measuring an outcome but a moment of connection and influence. We didn't sever ties in a misguided step toward avoidance or judgment. We honored our connection the best way we could while maintaining the necessary and healthy boundaries that allowed all of us to show up as our best selves at that time. In all those moments, love was shared between us, given and received.

It's important to honor those moments, too, because there is no real terminus where the mindful work can stop and families can return to an unexamined, easy, and automatic "normal." Recovery can and will have measurable gains worth celebrating, but the real investment isn't in the wins. The real investment is in showing up at each stop along the way on the family's recovery journey.

The following chapters explore five aspects of Parallel Recovery: Reflection, Psychoeducation, Communication and Behavior, Grief, and Self-Compassion.

I do not refer to these aspects of Parallel Recovery as "steps" because recovery is not a linear process with a beginning, middle, or end. Each of these aspects will instead weave continuously together to provide a framework for how to think about your own path toward healing, your role in the relationship with your person, and how to sustain and navigate the difficult realities of their substance use.

There is no one-size-fits-all set of steps or tricks that are guaranteed to lift someone out of substance use or fully protect you from how much this disorder sucks. But with thoughtful intention, honest patience, and a willingness to work on your patterns, you can take charge of your own healing. With these tools, you can ensure your personal recovery and offer your person the best possible chances.

PART ONE

PARALLEL RECOVERY

CHAPTER 1

HARD-EASY, EASY-HARD

IN 2012, my family and I were enjoying a beautiful summer in the Rockies, despite it being the hottest in my memory. I'm definitely a Colorado gal—I love the wide-open sky above the mountains and being outdoors. On that particular day, my kids had a swim meet, and our mountain bikes were loaded on the back of our car for some planned riding later in the day. As the swim meet was wrapping up, we started getting concerning text messages.

"Can you see the smoke from there?"

Some came with pictures attached showing a tall plume of smoke reaching up from the hillside where we lived. From the pictures, it was hard to see exactly how close it was to our neighborhood or grasp the size of the threatening gray cloud.

With the record heat and the previous dry spring, we knew wildfire was a concern and a possibility. I texted several people back, seeing if there was any specific news, but at that point, there wasn't much information beyond the presence of the plume on our hill. "I'm sure it's nothing," they said.

"Keep me updated!" I texted our friends back. We went on our planned mountain bike ride.

We just didn't know.

You can't always predict or be prepared for what's coming down the line that will completely throw your life in a new direction. We all have a picture in our heads of what we think our future should be; I certainly did. When you realize one day that a person you love is consumed by SUD, it can feel like that future has gone up in flames. You may feel like you woke up one day and poof, there it went, but it's not actually a quick burn. Sometimes, we try to hold on way too long to the way things were and the way things were supposed to be.

If I can just smother this flame, tamp it out, then things will be easy again.

When I work with families, there's a phrase I use early and often. It becomes a mantra of sorts, and it's a guiding question to help you take a good pause and consider the immediate choices in front of you.

Is this hard-easy? Or is this easy-hard?

When faced with a choice, the options are 1) to begin with the hard thing and then move on to the easier stuff (hard-easy) or 2) to begin with the easy thing and put off the hard (easy-hard). Notice that hard appears in both of those equations. Remembering this phrase shines a light on the reality of the available choices—none of this is going to be easy. When substance use is involved, there is no easy-easy option.

You can either do the hard thing—have the hard conversation, set the difficult boundary, feel the complicated grief that is coming, and start the work of changing your role in the equation—or you can put it off and choose something easier right now. You hope that things will work their way out, avoid the boundary for fear that they will be upset with you, and separate them from the reality of their situation because the consequences are just too painful for you to witness. Kick the hard can down the road.

On paper, this seems easier, but in practice, it's faking easy. The problem and its roots are still there, like a weed, waiting for the chance to emerge again. When you choose easy-hard, you end up holding your breath, hoping that the hard doesn't come. Or that, if you are quiet enough, it will miss you on its way by.

If they can just stop it, I won't have to do that hard thing.

If they don't come home drunk/high, I won't have to have this hard conversation.

If they can just get better, I won't need to grieve.

Holding your breath doesn't make the hard thing miss you; it just puts off the steps you need to take to face the problem and work it through. While you are holding your breath, your life is also passing you by.

When you understand and lean in to the *hard*, no matter what, you will be able to exhale on the other side. The hard will be done, and you can receive the ease earned from your work. Exhale, lean in, and learn to face the hard things now. Yes, you can.

If we are going to be honest, neither choice is truly easy. Hard is never fun, but I know that when you learn to lean in to the hard things, you will be able to exhale. There will be a sense of *less* hard on the other side of this difficult equation. You will feel relief that the thing you've been carrying around is now out there. You will feel empowered to understand that what you're expecting from yourself is to have your needs met too. It can be a scary unknown, the far side of the hard call, but there can also be a level of relief that you will never reach if you continue to hold your breath and kick the hard can down the road.

You have to exhale eventually.

⌒⌒

Later that summer day in 2012, we stowed the bikes again and headed back toward home. My phone, which had spotty service in that part of the mountains, reconnected with a few bars. Rapidly, it began to make panicked dinging sounds, sounds that I came to know quite well later when my son was in active addiction. Within a minute, I had a dozen updates from various friends and neighbors about the plume above our home on the hill.

They've told us to evacuate.

What's your garage code?

We need to evacuate.

We need to get in.

Never mind, the neighbor kid had it.

Your dog is with us. The photos from your walls are in my garage. I went in your jewelry drawer and grabbed shiny things.

We're evacuating.

Do you want us to get anything?

We sped home as fast as we could, and we made it in time to load up both cars with everything we could fit. With two small kids in tow, it wasn't much. The plume was bigger and closer than I thought. All up and down our street, people were looking up at the smoke cloud rising off the side of the mountain. Even that much closer, we couldn't see which way or how fast it was growing. It was hard to gauge how scared we should be. Everyone was just putting as much as they could in their cars without a clear strategy or plan.

At the end of the street, we had a community mailbox, the kind with locked boxes for each individual address. While the smoke rose up behind us on the hill, the mail person stoically went about his business, sorting the mail into each box. It was a funny juxtaposition, and I took a picture before driving away from the neighborhood.

My sons were very young that year, with my youngest a rising third grader and my eldest going into seventh that fall. We went to my mother's to stay and wait for more news. There was no way to know exactly how long it would be.

Helping my kids settle in, I opened my youngest son's suitcase to find it packed full of sweaters. It was the middle of the hottest summer, and we had evacuated away from a fire zone, yet my child had filled his suitcase full of sweaters, which he hated wearing even when it was cold enough for them. I asked him why he had only packed sweaters.

He shrugged at me. "I thought those were my nicest clothes."

It was an unprecedented situation for all of us. There was no guidebook or prioritized inventory of all the things in our home to reference. There was nothing to do but shake my head, laugh, and head to Target for something he could wear.

Years before the fire, I took my oldest son to his first day of first grade, walking him to his classroom and watching from the doorway with the other moms as the class got settled in. His teacher was a veteran, so the desks were set up in traditional rows. It was a corner classroom, brightly lit by windows along each wall. The teacher announced that all the students should find the desk with their name on it, sit down, and start on the worksheet on their desk.

My son loved learning, experiencing new things, talking with people, and exploring the world. He was full of questions. I watched him, adorably small and so cute with his striking dark hair, with hopes and plans for what would surely be an amazing life. The other kids in his class fell into compliance with the teacher's instructions, sat down at their desks, and began to fill in the worksheet. My son went to his desk, propped his foot on the chair, and just looked around him, taking in the classroom. I loved him for that too. His behavior made total sense to him.

As I took in that sight, I also saw that his behavior didn't make sense to others, especially his teacher. My instincts told me to get him out of that classroom. It wasn't the right place for him, and deep down, I felt it.

Except pulling him out would be so hard. I worked in education at the time and knew about classroom management and accommodations for different learning styles. Pulling him out would be a drastic, difficult step. It would mean massively changing our plans for daily life, facing criticisms from others who would disagree with the choice, and facing all my doubts about whether we could succeed at a new, untested plan.

So I didn't. I put aside that instinct and didn't listen to myself.

Within two weeks, he was coming home crying on a daily basis. It was the beginning of a long struggle with his school and his teachers. Eventually, we would learn about his dyslexia and find better places for him. Nothing ever came close to the comfort and ease that I saw on the other students' faces as they settled into what was clearly the right place for them.

I didn't think about that first day of first grade again until many years later, but when I think about it now, it was a lesson for me about hard-easy or easy-hard. I can't know whether pulling him out immediately would have been the right choice over the long term, but I do know that my instinct was correct—something wasn't right for him. That meant something hard was coming, and I wish I had understood that. I could either face it then or hold my breath and hope it would fix itself—the easy way.

⁂

After we initially evacuated the neighborhood, there were several days of waiting. The fire continued to burn. The neighborhood high school was used as a headquarters of sorts, and we gathered to get daily news briefs. The backdrop was perfect. On a good day, you could view the whole mountainside, including the ever-growing plume. We got used to the sight of it, and it seemed for a while that things were under control. We were given the okay to go into our neighborhood and collect more things from our homes. The fire hadn't been pushed back, but they said they were "holding" the fire. We'd have an hour, they said.

I was happy for the chance. It had become clear that the clothes we took were not sufficient, but even more so, I just needed to be in my space. There were so many unknowns, and I thought I would feel steadier being home, even for a very brief time. We all went back to the neighborhood. We had to check in with police there, who were acting partly as security and partly to keep track of how many were in the area.

I wanted to take care of my house, which I had been away from for what seemed like so long. I watered my plants, vacuumed, and wiped down the counters. For a little while, we were all just puttering, just being there in the house. The perception of normal felt "easy."

Again, we didn't know.

I was gathering some snacks and had just started thinking through what we should pack up when the doorbell rang. It was an officer. We needed to go. *Now.*

I protested that it hadn't been an hour—I had barely started. The officer was insistent, so we moved more quickly. I stopped taking mental inventory and started throwing what I could in kitchen trash bags. I told my sons that we had to go. My oldest son wanted to gather his awards and memorabilia from sports, but I told him we didn't have time. The officer helped us load our ski box onto the car, attaching it backward in his hurry.

I couldn't help but think, *What the hell?* It was not at all what I wanted. I needed the visit to give me a sense that things would be all right, let me be in my space where I was comfortable and could be reassured. I thought I'd have some time to regain some control and think things through, but instead, I had to tell my son to leave the things he wanted as we rushed back to the car. I turned the sprinkler on as we left, knowing it might not help but with no idea exactly how futile the situation really was.

There is news footage that shows how quickly the situation changed. The US Forest Service spokeswoman, Jerri Marr, was saying again what she'd been saying over and over: They were "holding" the fire back. No progress in putting it out, but it was relatively controlled. And then suddenly, the expression on the reporter's face changed. She saw people react to something behind her, and when she turned, that was it. No more "holding."

In a matter of minutes, things had changed, and the fire was surging forward. I couldn't believe how fast it moved. As we drove out of our neighborhood, our community was on fire. House after house went up in flames as we sped along the only road out of the area.

That was it. I had hoped for an easy. I never got it; I was in a hard.

All our instincts help us avoid getting hurt. When we love someone, we extend those instincts to them too. We do everything we can to keep them from getting hurt, even if the danger is a consequence of their own actions.

The consequences of the behavior and symptoms associated with SUD can be devastating. Often, the easy-hard choice is to try to intercept those consequences and lessen them however we can. We love our person and know that their behavior is being hijacked by the power of drugs and alcohol on the brain. Taking those things together, the easy thing is to bat away the consequences. Protect them from it so they stop getting hurt, and then we stop hurting by watching them hurt.

The world has a way of continuing to push consequences our way. Consider an oncoming asteroid. First spotted in the sky, it can appear tiny, like a fly that you can swat out of the way. But like asteroids, consequences also get bigger. They keep coming and growing, and eventually, they're not something you can absorb or bat away. If you've developed a pattern of deflecting the consequences over the course of years, they may even crush you both.

At first, the consequence seems small and manageable, like missing out on a trip or a slap on the wrist. But eventually, when left unaddressed or interfered with by you, those consequences get bigger and bigger. You are overwhelmed by the consequences, and your person is not even aware they have been happening.

The longer you choose easy-hard, the harder the hard will get.

That is not to say that once you do one hard thing, the rest of it is skipping through the daisies. Nor is it to say that you have to do all the hardest things imaginable immediately. It will take time. But avoiding hard is a choice, and that choice also has consequences.

Understanding the reality of the two choices—easy-hard or hard-easy—means accepting that hard stuff is coming. It's going to suck, and you can't just douse the flames or flick the asteroid out of the sky.

There is no easy-easy.

Telling yourself you can avoid the hard stuff is a comforting lie. In reality, you're just waiting for the day that you collapse because you cannot keep doing things this way. It's impossible to hold your breath forever.

What you can learn to do is make the hard sustainable. Stepping into the hard work is worth it, and it's doable. When you step into the hard work, you show your person that the hard work is possible and both of you are worth it. You can begin to live and thrive alongside the hard stuff. It will not look like what you had before all of this started, and it may not look like what you had in mind for yourself or them, but it will be real and honest, and that is where you get to exhale. That is your easy—finding peace and sustainability with what is.

After the fire took the neighborhood, there was more time in limbo as we tried to figure out whose home was destroyed and whose was spared. A friend who was a police officer sent us some pictures of our street. My husband and I puzzled over them. We couldn't even grab onto a landmark to judge what was what. It looked like the moon.

When we were able to return to the neighborhood, our whole side of the street was flattened. The other side of the street had houses standing, but ours—our home and everything in it—was gone. Right down to a heat-shattered foundation.

There is no easy, straight-line way to recover from a loss that profound. I tried to make it easy by telling myself that it was just stuff—my family was okay. And that *is* what mattered. I silver-lined the situation. But it didn't account for the impact it had on all of us and how deeply that change would be felt for years and years to come.

I told my children that it was all going to be okay. My youngest fully believed me because if Mom said it was going to be okay, then, of course, it was going to be okay. My oldest understood, perhaps for the first time, that I couldn't actually control everything enough to make that guarantee. The unspoken message I gave in these untruths was that I didn't believe he could handle the hardship. Or maybe it was that I couldn't handle watching him experience it.

We were able to get a rental place within walking distance of where we were rebuilding. Most of the neighborhood came back to rebuild, but it took a long time. It took us fourteen months and nine days to finally settle the insurance claim. The process of rebuilding was complicated and surreal. There were so many moving parts between the contractors, the insurance, and the city. It was more than a full-time job to coordinate, and there was always some new element that would come up and have to be dealt with.

One day, for example, the city informed us that they had scheduled the "metal removal day." So contractors had to be informed when the metal would be collected from the debris and destruction so they could plan accordingly. Nothing about the process seemed to be a straight line.

People helped, both individuals and the collective community. People gave money and used items, and the lunch at the children's school was free for the next year for those who had lost their homes in the fire. It was vital support but, emotionally, a poor replacement for a home.

The emotional impact would come up in response to what might seem like the smallest things. An acquaintance offered us a set of dishes they didn't use anymore, but I didn't want them. I wanted the kind that I had, that I had chosen and loved and used every day. I never wanted to seem ungrateful for the help or dismissive of the privilege I had in being able to rebuild. But none of the help could take away the profound emotional impact that came with being so violently displaced from the home we had made.

My son could feel this too. By the time my oldest was in seventh grade, we had long ago established accommodations to help with his dyslexia. In some ways, this helped him at school, but it also set him apart. He didn't want to be seen as different. Now, every Friday after the fire, he was one of the kids sent home with a suitcase full of food. It was one of the clumsier ways the community tried to help. We could get food—what we didn't have was T-shirts, a spaghetti strainer, wedding photos, and dozens of other things that we couldn't think to ask for until we reached for them and remembered they were gone.

We would spend years replacing and making do and getting by. A year or two after the fire, my son wrote an essay for school he titled "A House on Top of a Home." The physical task of rebuilding was all-consuming, and it left very little time for us to just sit and feel the loss and process it emotionally. What we were left with was a gradual replacement of our things and the raising of a house where we once had a home. It was pain that we glossed over with paint.

It is uncomfortable to sit with something painful.

When someone is struggling with SUD, they are in pain. Their very nervous system is working against them. It is hard to sit in discomfort with someone who is experiencing that level of pain. It feels easier to detach and walk away, or to lecture about why the situation needs to change, or to lay out authoritative plans on how you're going to "fix" the person. But our instinct to reach for those easy actions only puts off the hard stuff.

It's hard, instead, to step into those moments with your person and acknowledge how difficult this is for them, how much it sucks, and to listen to how they are feeling in that moment, regardless of whether we understand their choices or behavior. It's important to create a space where you can coexist with them—safely, as they exist now—in this painful struggle.

This does *not* mean that you become part of the logistical support that allows them to continue using or that you participate in their problem. You can't bat away the asteroid of the consequences that might occur for them. But you can find the space between protecting your peace and closing the door on them.

Pain and dysregulation in the nervous system can be like that wildfire up on the hill, giving off that ominous plume of smoke. We see it, and our first instinct is to tamp down that fire. But tamping it down doesn't work.

Have you ever watched a wildfire rage on TV and asked, "Why don't they just pour water on that thing?" It feels like you could just smother it somehow as it crawls along the forest floor. Every fire you've ever known has worked that way—douse it with water, deprive it of oxygen, or take away its fuel, and it will fizzle out. Easy.

Those are our instincts when we see a fire from afar. But wildfires are different. You understand that fully when you see one up close. It spreads along the ground, moving like something living. It exudes massive heat that you can feel in the wind when it turns your way. Wildfires burn at between 1000-2000°F, which is not like any other fire. It melts metal. It won't be smothered by a blanket or quenched by a bucket of water.

When you're faced with a wildfire up close where you can see the reality of it, it becomes clear that's not how it works. When you try to tamp it out, force it down in some quick and expedient way, it just flares back up again twice as high. It has to burn itself out. Fighting a wildfire is about holding the line and protecting what you can. To protect population-dense areas and structures, they dig in cuts along the hillside, attempting to create boundaries that the fire might follow. Sometimes, the fire jumps the boundary, and they have to find a new way to lessen its damage. And sometimes, there's nothing they can do.

To this day, I can still see the scars along the hillside in my neighborhood where the firefighters carved ditches to try to contain the flames. I remember, when we were first allowed to visit the remains of the neighborhood after its destruction, that the firefighters were still there. Many wept openly. "We tried," they told us. "We tried so hard."

The work of recovery, for both those struggling with SUD and their families, is hard. But you can do hard things. You can survive hard things. And you can rebuild.

CHAPTER 2

SHARING THE BURDEN OF CHANGE

I HEARD a parable once that comes to me often. It's Hasidic in origin, but there are many variations. It goes something like this:

There once was a king (Isn't there always a king?) who ruled over a land the best that he could. He cherished his family, but just as his son was growing into a young man, the son began to embarrass him in front of the kingdom. (The parable is a bit light on the details here, but I imagine him drinking too much wine, making impulsive decisions, and generally just behaving boorishly.)

The king and his son argued, and things got heated. The king banished his son from the kingdom. (Perhaps the king was bluffing, assuming that under this threat of banishment, the son would see how badly he was misbehaving and come back under the king's control as he had always done as a child. Or perhaps the king saw only two options: Make his son change or banish him.) So, the son left the kingdom.

As time passed, the king began to regret his decision. His anger cooled, and soon, he realized that missing his child hurt him much more than any embarrassment his son's actions could cause him.

He called his messengers and told them to go and find his son and tell him to come back home.

But they came back without him.

His son had refused his invitation. The servants couldn't compel him to come back; he was living elsewhere, and his hurt and bitterness were too strong to just return home at the king's calling.

The king's plan didn't work because he was trying to force change on another person without acknowledging his role in the greater problem and without validating the experience of banishment that his son certainly felt. The son's actions were fully his own, but so were the king's. Every one of the king's reactions was a choice—the heated argument, the displays of anger, the demands for change, and, eventually, the banishment. When he sent his servants out to retrieve his son, the king had changed his mind but not his strategy. He was still trying to force the outcome he believed he needed. The result was to strain the relationship even more.

We all have needs that must be met for us to live happy, full lives. Those needs are physical, emotional, and psychological. Sometimes, we reach for something to fulfill a need without realizing that it will only provide temporary satisfaction; in the long run, it will cause more harm than good. The more we reach for these surface-level solutions, the more habitual our reach becomes. Eventually, if we continue to reach for band-aid solutions, we forget we even have a cut. Our focus turns to the band-aids themselves and the need for them to remain in place for us to feel safe.

This cycle is part of the core pattern of substance use. Someone consumes drugs or alcohol as a way to fill a need—calming anxiety, dulling physical pain, or self-medicating to numb myriad pains. Over time, the substance becomes a stand-in for the need itself until the need and the self-medication become nearly impossible to disentangle on one's own. It develops into a disorder that hijacks the decision-making process.

But this cycle of confusing needs with self-medicating behaviors can become a trap for anyone, with or without substance use. When our person is enveloped in substance use, it's like we're standing on the outside looking in. Watching their destructive behavior hurts. We experience a powerful need to ease the pain—to fix the situation. Our natural and understandable reaction is to try to force our person to change.

But our needs belong to us. They are our burden, our heavy coats to wear. We are not on the outside, looking in. We are a part of a greater situation, one that has become unsustainable and needs to change for our well-being.

When we say, *I* need *them* to change so *I* can feel better and be at peace, we're putting our heavy coat on our person. But our person already has their own heavy coat. Forcing our burden on them is neither fair nor effective.

This process is difficult because the impulse to fix things isn't "wrong," exactly. The situation does need to change. SUD doesn't spring from nowhere. It doesn't occur in a vacuum. It's a symptom of a greater issue. We all carry a piece of that greater problem, and that problem can only be healed by healing the connections we have with each other.

If we can acknowledge our own needs, how those needs have influenced our actions, and the role we have played in the whole problem, we can move toward change. If not, we get stuck—we try to control the entire situation ourselves, imposing our needs and burdens onto the people we love. We proverbially send out the messengers to bring our prince home.

The messengers come back empty-handed every time, and we are disappointed.

What the king failed to realize—what so many of us overlook— is that control is not love. Trying to force someone to change is simply not an expression of love. And because it's not rooted in love, it's almost always ineffective. Constantly pushing our person and making all the important choices on their behalf won't lead them through recovery. It is an expression of control that doesn't work.

It's understandable that we want to control the situation. Watching your person go through these issues is scary. But trying to control someone else's behavior is ineffective, no matter how scary it is. Dedicating all your power to attempts at control will never steer you closer to the solution. It will only drive you—and them—further away from healing.

Imagine a crying child, say around twelve years old. Their tears and wails are intense. They say, "This is the worst day of my life." We know better. We can see better. We can understand better. Or at least, we think we can. So, we try to shape *their* reactions according to *our* experiences. We ask someone else to react based not on what they have experienced but on what we have.

With only twelve years of experience under their belts, they have a very different perspective. This day may, in fact, be the worst day of their life. That's huge! They need to feel the big emotions that understandably come with the worst experience they can remember feeling.

It would be incredibly insensitive to say, "Calm down. Be quiet. You're twelve. You're going to have worse days." It doesn't matter whether we know that to be true or not. When we say "Be quiet," we are saying, "Don't experience that." We are teaching them that their feelings are too big for us to accommodate, and they should tuck them away somewhere. They should make their emotions smaller. When people aren't given the opportunity to experience big things in a safe environment—when they don't have the space to process intense things and integrate them into their total human experience —they develop maladaptive coping skills, like lashing out in anger, isolating themselves, or numbing their pain with substances.

Our urge to control the experience is understandable. But it can be incredibly destructive. It is not love.

So what's the alternative? Empowerment.

Empowerment is love.

When we seize complete control and responsibility, we actively take power away from our person. When we truly focus on empowerment, we demonstrate that change is possible.

Imagine that same twelve-year-old with the tear-streaked face and dramatic wails. As is often the case with kids, a few months later, they experience an entirely new "worst day of their life." What if, instead of wanting to control their behavior by telling them to be quiet, we allow them to undergo the pain of this experience? What if we sat with them, creating a safe connection and space to experience the "worst day of their life"? What if we let them cry until their tears are spent and their wails are exhausted? What if we said, "I can see how hard that was, and I'm so sorry. I also know you are strong enough to feel this and be okay."

Sitting through a child's pain is hard. It's uncomfortable and takes an enormous amount of self-control. It's much easier to say, "I know better than you, so be quiet," because in that moment, the outcome we think we want is for the crying to stop.

The easy solution—forcing the crying to stop—does not address the child's root need in the moment. It's the easy-hard solution because the crying is only a symptom of the pain. When we force the symptom to stop, we push the emotional experience down the pike, which undoubtedly makes the pain more intense when it eventually resurfaces.

For the same reason, saying "stop using drugs" doesn't work. The substance use we're trying to stop is a symptom. It's serving a need that the person has no other tools to satisfy, and until they do the work of learning how to experience and serve their root needs, the symptom will keep emerging—over and over—because the *need* will keep emerging over and over.

We can't do that work for them. We can only give them an emotionally safe space to do that work. We can only tell them that we can see how hard this is, AND we also know that they are strong enough to do it. We can adjust our responses from controlling to empowering. We can participate in the process of changing rather than continuing to participate in the problem.

By changing our reactions to responses, we can show that change is possible. Our person needs to see that. But first, we must step up and work on ourselves. We must look inward and honestly examine who we have become in reaction to this painful situation. In our worry and our fear, have we become the type of person to search through someone else's things? To monitor them in every way we can and mistrust anything and everything they say? Have we become the type of person who tries to control the behavior of others in order to get our needs met? Have we become reactionary and quick to anger, withholding love in hopes of reaching a transactional agreement?

Every family's circumstances are different, so the specific way you'll approach these changes is an individual question. Regardless of the details, the process of change for everyone can begin with an honest reflection of who we are right now. We can do the work to see ourselves clearly, why we do what we do, and understand our root needs. We can slow down and choose our actions with intention. We can start to break the cycle of participating in the problem with our reactionary choices and start to be a part of the recovery process by responding with intention, compassion, and love.

In my own family's struggle with SUD, we, like countless other families, tried many things that did not work—for any of us. It took a long time for the tides to shift and for things to gradually get truly better. Part of that shift started when I realized that I had to do something different—but that meant that *I* had to start the work toward change in myself.

While my son was going through treatment, my husband and I attended a family program. During a mirroring exercise, my family members were asked to describe one another by stepping into the others' shoes. My husband was asked to step into my role and introduce me. He said, "My name is Lisa, and I like things just so." From there, he went on to describe me with a level of accuracy that only a husband of many years could have. The group laughed; I did not.

It hurt me to hear myself depicted like that, and it took a long time and lots of reflection to understand why I felt the exercise so deeply. While I couldn't deny that his description was correct, it wasn't who I wanted to be in my family.

I realized that I had allowed this disorder to change me—I had become someone who micromanaged, controlled, and scripted life. I had perceived my control as helpful, believing that I was creating a safe space for my family.

I wanted so badly to give us all somewhere safe, where we could exist together and support one another. I wanted them to be able to put down their shackles and express themselves. I wanted it so much that I had been trying to manufacture it. And in trying to force a safe space through my control, I had created the opposite.

To create an emotionally safe space means allowing people to exist fully as themselves—it means including them as they are today, whatever that looks like. Instead, I had been saying, "You are going to be included by sitting here, listening to this, and saying that." I thought that was inclusion. But when I reflected, I realized that I was not allowing my son to experience and share his life. Completely against my own intentions, I was making spaces unsafe. I was participating in the problem.

And that is part of why my control strategy was not working. I wasn't providing space for my son to experience his life and recover and grow; I was taking up space. My own need to see progress was guiding all my communication choices, and as a result, I was participating in the problem by adding to my son's burden. He was carrying my heavy coat, my need for things to be a certain way. Not only was I asking him to get better for himself, but I was trying to force him to get better *for me*. He had to solve his pain and mine too.

That wasn't fair. It wasn't a good way forward for any of us. He had his own heavy winter coat. He didn't have the strength to carry mine too.

Over time, I came to understand that my burden is mine and his burden is his. This seemingly simple concept created a huge shift in how I thought about the problem. It became a new guiding light for my choices. It wasn't easy; it required changing my perspective on my responsibility to myself and my family. I had to learn to let go of control and practice self-compassion.

Like releasing control, self-compassion is hard. That's why we so often default to self-pity. We justify and validate our behaviors in ways that feel good to us in the moment.

I didn't start the problem.

This is happening to me.

I am the injured party here.

But healing isn't concerned with how things started, only with where they are. Insisting on how things started and looking for blame, explanation, and causality will interfere with you loving and accepting yourself and your person as you and they are today.

Self-pity is the easy-hard choice. When we dig down to find a root cause somewhere outside ourselves, we are taking the simpler path. It's easier to place blame externally than to accept the reality of the situation and the way we're participating in it at that moment.

Self-compassion, on the other hand, is the hard-easy choice. Self-compassion requires recognizing the gap between how you are actually being experienced and how you want to be experienced. It requires acknowledging that you are the only one who can fix that gap and that it is your burden to bear.

You can recognize that gap with compassion and empathy for yourself. You can work to understand what need you thought you were filling with your decisions. You can forgive yourself for the choices you would make differently now. You can reflect on how you can make better ones. You can create a safe space for yourself to grow. You can acknowledge that this has been hard, and it is understandable that you have been reactive.

You can start to do that work even in the context of your person's continuing SUD because your recovery is what you need. You can begin to recover whether or not *their* behavior has changed.

It's hard work. It requires accepting vulnerability and fallibility. But you can do that hard work. You are strong enough to do that hard work, and you will get even stronger and healthier. You will become a model of change for your person, demonstrating through your growth that the process is possible. It can work. Your growth and your connection with the person you hold space for can become part of their guiding light toward recovery too.

Sharing the burden of change is not about trying to carry your person's burden. Taking on others' work is not loving or compassionate. It's self-harm. If we let it, SUD can pull others down, multiplying the damage and the hurt—two-for-one or three, four, five-for-one. It can manifest in ways that are not easy to see when we're in the thick of things.

For one family member I worked with, the impulse to control and carry has manifested in genuine physical pain. Her son has been in the thralls of SUD for over two decades, and she has fought hard to pull him back from it. The stress from such a long period of ongoing trauma has raised her cortisol levels and kept them high, resulting in chronic illness and pain. She is not the one with SUD, but his illness is entangled in hers just as much as she is entangled in his.

Sharing the burden of change means being willing to identify which of your core needs aren't being met by your actions and reactions and discovering the changes you need to make in order to be healthy and strong for your relationship and yourself.

Our person's recovery cannot depend on ours. And our recovery cannot depend on theirs.

By identifying which part of the burden is ours to carry—and then owning that part—we model growth, accountability, and healing. We become a living example of what the necessary work looks like by taking steps for our recovery and resisting the urge to place our recovery burden on someone who is struggling with their own challenges.

There's more to recovery than your person's healing. And there's more to the parable of the king than the banishment.

After the king's messengers came back empty-handed, the king thought about his son for a long time. Sometimes, he got angry again, but mostly, he just missed his son terribly. He realized he could not force the outcome that he wanted, but neither could he sit and do nothing.

So he asked his messengers to take him to the place where they had found his son. He wanted to be with his son, wherever he was. At first, the prince wouldn't even look at him. He refused to even turn in the direction of home.

Still, the king sat with his son. He told him that he understood that the prince couldn't return to the kingdom. He told him he understood why he could not face home. Finally, the king said what he'd come to say. "I will meet you here when I am able," he said. "Until you are ready to turn around."

CHAPTER 3

ALIGNING VALUES

IF YOU ENVISION your life as a car, who is driving? Our root needs are a major driving force in our lives, but left on their own, they are not necessarily good navigators.

When we feel desperate to protect our loved person, fear often steps forward to drive the car. Decisions guided by fear at the wheel are naturally reactionary, impulsive, and ineffective. When we want to protect ourselves and respond to the discomfort we're feeling, anger may try to take the wheel—but anger isn't much better at driving than fear. When anger drives our actions, we engage in power struggles, lash out, and cause further harm to our already strained relationships.

We cannot completely rid ourselves of fear and anger. But we can direct them into the back seat, acknowledging their presence but asking them to stop guiding the way. When you're confronted with painful situations, navigating them takes reflection and carefully formed, intentional choices. That means you need your true self—the most authentic version of yourself—to be in the driver's seat.

How do you find that core self? How do you activate and

empower that version of yourself to be in charge, especially when things are difficult? To be sure that your true self is driving the car, you need to reflect inward and identify your core values and how they have influenced your decisions and responses in your life, family, and relationship with your person.

Those core values are the foundational pillars of who you are, what you care most about in your life, and—perhaps most importantly—how you want to be experienced by those around you. They are the thumbprint you leave on your relationships. With our values in alignment, we can then begin to reflect on whether our actions and behavior are being received as expressions of that core value—or as something else that we did not intend.

When families commit to exploring and rediscovering their values and intentions, they can learn how to reengage in their relationships aligned with those intentions while using effective and compassionate communication tools. Being part of the solution requires identifying what values you need to hold up as your North Star, knowing how you want others to experience you, and striving to always engage with them in that way—regardless of their reactions.

The North Star has been a symbol of guidance for centuries. The North Star doesn't show you the whole map of the terrain, but it points to a destination. When you keep your eye on your North Star, each step you take might not be exactly where you want to go, but it won't take you astray.

This is true of your core values too. They serve as a tool throughout this process, so it's important to begin by defining them —your North Star—and checking in along the way so you can make sure you're headed in the right direction, even when it feels like you are lost.

When beginning this process, some families get stuck in an outcome-oriented mindset. They can react to this step of the process with impatience. There is a desire to "fix" their person, save them from the pattern of behavior that has them trapped—*now*. But as we discussed in the previous chapter, it is ineffective to force change on others.

At this stage, you need to recognize the pattern of behavior that has *you* trapped. You may not be the one struggling with SUD, but if everything you've done to try to solve the problem has not only failed to reach your desired external outcome but continuously made you feel worse and more helpless, then you are also stuck in a pattern that is not working for you. If your life has become unmanageable, you need to find a new way to manage it.

The solution to this pain may seem simple to you: Your person must recover from their SUD. But when we accept that we cannot force that outcome, we can step back and take in what we want in a broader picture. What do you hope for from your life and for your family greater than your person stopping what they are doing? What do you want to be the guiding light for your choices, not through to the "end" of this struggle, but forever?

When we are feeling stuck in a painful situation, it is easy to dream of its conclusion—an end to this discomfort. We tell ourselves that as soon as this is over, the rest will be easy. We can exhale and take our iced tea out to the porch and just exist in that state of perpetual ease.

This is a fantasy. We have to release it. There is no real end to discomfort—life tends to throw things at us, and no monumental, singular effort on our part can stop that forever.

So, we need to embrace a different, achievable outcome: Living in alignment with our values. Our values represent who we want to be with others and for ourselves, both at ease *and* when confronted with discomfort. When we do the reflective work of identifying our values and honoring them with our words and behaviors, we will be better prepared to enjoy the joyful times of life and weather the difficult times with grace.

Imagine yourself in your dotage, and in those twilight years, imagine you could gather around you all the people from your life. If they were to reflect on their lives with you, what would you want them to say? How would you want your legacy to be reflected in their memory of you? What kind of parent, sibling, friend, or partner do you want to be remembered as?

Perhaps you want to be remembered for your devotion to your loved ones, your welcoming persona, your joyful sense of humor, your generosity, your unshakable faith, your steadfast responsibility, your creativity, or any number of positive attributes we may try to embody.

This bittersweet exercise can show us two things—it can reveal our core values, and it can shine a light on whether we are really expressing those values. It can help us see whether we are living our values in a way that is felt and experienced by others.

It has been said that any time two people meet, there are actually six people present, for both have who they see themselves to be, who the other sees them to be, and who they really are. The further apart those three versions of each person are, the more potential for confusion, conflict, and pain. When you reflect on how you would want to be remembered in the future by those who know you, ask yourself honestly how they would describe you *now*.

Perhaps they would remember everything you did for them or every time you stepped in and got them out of trouble. Perhaps they would remember all the meals you prepared and the financial support you gave. Most of us hope for something deeper in our loved ones' memories. Rather than a list of services rendered, we want to be remembered by how we expressed our core values.

If all we needed to live these values was intention, the process would be easy. But intention isn't the only thing that influences our behavior—we also have a complex set of needs and emotions. The way we are received and experienced by others might not be the best expression of these values. It might actually be an expression of how our values collide with our unmet needs and unregulated emotions.

When I heard my husband say, "I am Lisa, and I want things just so," it was painful. I had been trying to *force* a safe, inclusive space, not realizing that my approach was antithetical and impossible. My core value was inclusivity, so I wanted people in my circle to feel safe in my spaces and in my home. I wanted everyone to feel comfort in the way I communicated with them.

But until my needs were met and my emotions were regulated, it was impossible to express my values in a way that would resonate the way I wanted them to. Instead, my family was experiencing the shadow side of my core values.

Every core value has a shadow side. The shadow side of my value of inclusivity was the origin of my instinct for control. While I wanted to express my desire for inclusivity, I also needed safety, security, and peace. I meant well, but because I hadn't really considered how my actions and communication choices were being received and felt, I wasn't able to think beyond myself. I was blinded to my effect on those around me. In the end, I was neither serving my values nor my root needs.

Other values have their shadow side as well. The value of humor can be a wonderful thing. Laughter shared among people can lift spirits and create genuine connection through that shared moment of humor and emotional resonance. But humor can also be used to separate and cause little cuts of harm. We typically call this sarcasm. Sarcasm is the humor that bites back because we feel threatened or unheard. When we use humor in self-defense, we deepen hurt feelings and antagonism within our circle rather than creating that sense of unified understanding through shared laughter. Both humor and sarcasm come from the same root instinct—and if we do not stop to consider which face of that value is showing up with us, our positive intentions will not be felt by those around us.

Being a steadfast and responsible family provider is a worthy goal and an admirable quality. But in remembering you, would your person say that your steadfast responsibility was an example for them? Or would they list all the things you helped them pay for? Financial stability is something we should aim to teach by example, not take on as a mantle to bear forever. Especially if providing that financial stability for someone who is hurting themselves through substance use prevents them from ever feeling the real consequences of that behavior.

It can be hard to see how a value like devotion to our loved ones could have a shadow side. But the shadow side of many values can be found in the ways they harm us. Devotion seems like absolute love. Many of the families I work with identify devotion as their core value. But even this loving value needs to be examined critically when we consider how it is being experienced by those we are devoted to.

How would your person describe the legacy of your devotion? A list of all the ways you sacrificed yourself and your life fails to describe a legacy of devotion. Through this exercise, we can really see that all of those things you do through devotion can evaporate over time. If you showed devotion by always having the doors to your home available, you sacrificed your peace for a temporary solution for your person. If you always provided the cash needed to bail them out of the consequences of their behavior, then you sacrificed your security to give them a temporary solution.

If your value of devotion leads you to being a doormat, to never saying no, to giving constantly through your pain all that you have over and over, then the legacy of your devotion is one of self-harm. Self-sacrifice is not a value we want to model for others to emulate.

Whether your legacy is to be inclusive, a provider, funny and full of joy, devoted, or something else, truly embodying your values means modeling what they look like in a healthy person. If we want our values to be central to our legacies—and if we want those legacies to be uplifting, rich, and a model for our loved one—we cannot simply express them in whatever way feels easiest at the time. We must reflect on how those values serve others *and* how they serve us.

Once you have committed to an honest reflection of how your values may be experienced by those around you, you can also begin to see your own needs more holistically and consider how you can express your values while also ensuring your well-being.

Life is complicated, so a healthy life is one that accounts for the different shades of need everyone shares. There are a few different ways of describing these needs, and I prefer the eight dimensions of wellness model. This model describes eight mutually codependent spheres of well-being: emotional, physical, occupational, social, spiritual, intellectual, environmental, and financial. Within these spheres, there's a natural give and take. When they are all being considered and protected, they can help regulate each other and compensate when circumstances weaken one area or another.

For instance, it's clear that when we are well-supported socially, spiritually, intellectually, and environmentally, we recover more easily from something like a major financial loss or a physical illness. We can often find evidence of this by looking at those in our lives who seem able to easily bounce back compared to those who don't. Over time, if one or more dimensions are consistently neglected, our entire system of needs cannot work as well to support each other. Our health suffers. Destabilizing circumstances have longer and more difficult repercussions. We experience a much lower quality of life.

You cannot be of help to a person struggling when your own needs are unstable and strained past the point of sustainability. To support the possibility of your person's recovery, you must be well in yourself. Part of what this requires in practice is to find ways to protect your wellness—all eight dimensions—while maintaining your loving connection to your person.

This is not a contradiction.

You *can* express your values and have them be felt in the way you intend them to be felt. You *can* maintain your connection to your person where they are right now *and* care for your well-being. You *can* love your person as they are, separate from and regardless of the pattern of destructive behavior they are trapped in.

This will likely require a change of perspective and habits. It will require making different choices and using different strategies than the ones you've been using.

In later chapters, we'll explore different strategies for communicating with your person, setting functional boundaries, and building that connection in ways that protect your wellness. However, there is no singular magic set of words that you can memorize and recite like a script to set these boundaries. After all, echoing someone else only makes you sound like someone else, and that is not a path toward a genuine connection to your person. The right way to manage this balance is dependent on your situation, your values, your history with your person, and the connection you want to have with them.

All the strategies through the later chapters of this book will ask you to consider both your values and your wellness. We use these frameworks to empower you to analyze your situation and develop reliable decision-making guides. Before you can use them as your North Star, you need to recognize and acknowledge the gap between how you are presenting yourself to those around you and how you want to be received. All of this reflection takes some time, and that requires taking a moment to *pause*. A pause doesn't feel like a crucial thing to do; rather, it feels like doing nothing at all. But from what we understand about psychology, the pause is essential.

Viktor Frankl was an Austrian neurologist, psychiatrist, and Holocaust survivor. In his book *Man's Search for Meaning*, he chronicles his experiences in Nazi concentration camps and outlines his psychological approach, which emphasizes finding purpose and meaning in life, even in the face of suffering. Frankl developed the field of logotherapy. Unlike other forms of psychotherapy that may emphasize pleasure or power, logotherapy posits that finding purpose and meaning in life is essential for psychological health. He argued that self-definition is an important aspect of psychological well-being. A cycle of struggle and trauma can make people feel trapped in a loop of simply reacting to their environment, leading to feelings of emptiness and existential frustration.

Frankl recognized, like many scholars of the human mind before him, that our brain reacts to stimuli in the same way our whole nervous system does. When you touch a hot stove, you jerk your hand back. You don't stop to consider the heat or the potential for a burn. The same is true when your doctor taps your patellar tendon with a reflex hammer—the jerk of the knee happens in the very next instant.

Our brains can work the same way—the instinct of response can be immediate. The neurochemical fight-or-flight response can be triggered in a snap of the fingers without any time to consider the stimulus, let alone our core values or emotional needs.

Describing his understanding of Frankl's views, author Steven Covey said, "Between stimulus and response there is a space. In that space is our power to choose our response. In our response lies our growth and our freedom."

That gap between the stimulus and our response is a place for us to pause. We can harness that gap to take control of our brains and make decisions about our outward responses. This space or pause allows us to shift from reacting to responding.

That gap is not necessarily a comfortable place to be. In fact, it is often marked by profound discomfort. When we experience something acutely, we want to ease the discomfort as quickly as possible. In those cases, our brains turn to an immediate reaction. But we can learn to take a pause before our reaction and extend that space, that pause. We can use that time to formulate a thoughtful response that reflects who we want to be in the world.

To make space for thoughtfulness and choice, we must learn how to sit in the discomfort of the pause. The fast pace and immediacy of our culture has lowered our tolerance level for discomfort, but growth and development do not come without it. If we want to become the people of our legacies, we need to develop the ability to respond with mindfulness rather than letting our first automatic reaction out of the gate unchecked.

In the pause is freedom. It allows us to escape the cycle of reactionary behavior that can trap us. That freedom is also our responsibility to take up. We are responsible for finding and shaping the meaning of our lives because no one else can.

When you deliberately hold fast to your values and understand how their shadow sides might lead you astray, you can put yourself back in the driver's seat. Fear, anger, self-doubt, and pain can take the back seat. We acknowledge that they are there, but they no longer guide us. By now, you know you can't will away this hurt and fear. Discomfort will be part of this journey, but we can learn how to manage that discomfort and keep control of the wheel.

A person with SUD also has that pause, though the disorder makes it even harder and more uncomfortable. The disorder can transform that discomfort into pain that feels like life or death. Their addiction is driving the car of their lives, and taking back the wheel will take support, time, and work.

But if we can model what taking control of the car looks like—using that space between stimulus and response to make mindful, values-based choices that allow us to take hold of our lives—we can support them in doing the same.

CHAPTER 4

FAMILY PATTERNS

WE ARE MORE INTERTWINED with our families than many of us realize or perhaps would like to admit. Their scars impact us because we love and care deeply for them, but we are also intertwined by our circumstances.

We exist as close points in the greater web of cause and effect that has brought us to this moment. Family patterns can be passed down to us through expectations, financial obligations and habits, social pressures, and even the expression of our very genetic code. Strategies and coping mechanisms also get passed down and shared within families. These coping mechanisms may no longer serve us, and the more we learn, the more we can see how these strategies interfere with effective and healthy ways of dealing with conflict, mental illness, and unhealthy behaviors such as substance use.

The phrase "creatures of habit" speaks to the nature of habit only partly accurately because habits seem like things we do without examination or thought. Habits are creature actions, reactions we carry out without consulting our higher-thinking selves. Habits can be beneficial, like stretching upon rising or drinking a full glass of water at lunchtime. Habits can also keep us trapped in unhelpful reactive patterns, especially in how we communicate with each other, handle conflict, and try to help in ineffective ways.

Habits are ingrained by repetition and a deep-seated belief in their effectiveness, which carves deeper into their groove with each pass. These grooves can be beneficial paths of ease through bracken —the repeated action of feet preventing the growth of new obstacles in the path. Or they can be like a rope dug into the skin that forms scar tissue.

But habits and family patterns can be adjusted and remade in better ways. It's not easy. It starts with an honest reflection on what those patterns are, where they might come from, and how they have served us in the past.

As discussed in the previous chapter, it's hard to hear that the first step is to stop and think. Slowing down to identify your core values and your family's patterns can feel maddeningly passive when it feels like your person is in crisis.

When we're trapped in a pattern, it can feel like we need to act immediately, choose quickly, or insist harder until something changes. But recognizing the pattern and making a choice to step out of the cycle that no longer serves you in not being inactive—it's not passive. It's a deliberate step toward something better.

Family dynamics can be complicated and fraught with tensions from opposing needs and scars, either from past trauma or simply a history of complicated family experiences. What starts as an instinct to love and protect can often be expressed as control and mistrust, deepening rather than healing the conflict and tension.

Complicating this even further, our family dynamics also exist inside of us. The concept of Internal Family Systems acknowledges that we are made up of different parts that take on different roles and behaviors to fulfill different needs.

Have you ever felt frozen in indecision? Part of you wants one thing, part of you wants something else entirely, and you feel stuck between the two options. This type of internal conflict happens because we all genuinely contain multiple perspectives. The mind is naturally multifaceted because this allows us to weigh and counterbalance different needs.

Just like families, the various aspects of our whole selves can be in conflict, but they can also have different relationships to one another. Often, in times of challenge, aspects of ourselves develop a sense of protectiveness—even overprotectiveness—of other aspects. Parts of us adamantly resist allowing other parts to change and grow because how we have been doing things has kept us emotionally protected in the past. When this dynamic occurs, we can get stuck in patterns of protectiveness that lead to destructive behaviors.

All the parts of you are good and necessary, but some parts of you may carry burdens that they need help putting down. Those burdens may be pain from your past or burdens passed between or along from others.

When communicating with your family and loved ones, it's important to understand what part of *you* is speaking and acting, and what part of *them* is speaking and acting. Which part is really showing up in this interaction? When we are dysregulated and out of harmony with ourselves, parts of us will seek out ways to be protective of the vulnerable, wounded, and struggling parts of us.

That same internal disconnection exists in our loved ones struggling with SUD. For them, the protection they seek out may come in the form of substance use. Using substances can ease the pain and keep the vulnerable part hidden, and it "protects" the part of our person that carries that pain. Beyond a certain point, substance use becomes the whole solution. There can be a million forms of struggle underneath the substance use—isolation, complex trauma, a stunted need for community, or even just the deeply held belief that they're not "fun" without the substance. It can lead to scary behavior, and that feeds into the distraction that the substance use serves.

When we react to that scary behavior with attempts to control and force change, we are also being hijacked by an over-protective part of ourselves that disconnects rather than connects to our person. In these circumstances, we aren't communicating with our person or their pain. We're communicating with the behavior of substance use. The substance use becomes a shield for that wounded, vulnerable inner part of our person. Bashing that shield with our own only plays into the strategy and perpetuates the cycle of behavior.

By looking at ourselves and identifying which part of us is showing up, we can learn to speak and behave differently. We can learn to communicate with the part of the person who's hurting and work toward developing an emotionally safe space for healing.

The vulnerable part of ourselves and our person can be thought of as an inner child. The emotional pain that the vulnerable part feels may be a real remembered trauma from childhood, it might be a cultural or social burden that no longer serves a need, or it might be something else entirely. No matter the source, the emotional pain feels like a continuous attack because it has not been faced, felt, and dealt with in a healthy way.

The hurt is not going to go away by being pushed into a corner. We can create the space to do that for ourselves and our person by slowing down to stop, think, and reflect. It may feel like we're at war, but when part of that battle is happening on the inside, we have to look inward and create peace by understanding why we are reacting that way before we can help others do the same. To create peace within, we need to understand where those burdens came from and how we can gently put them down.

~~~

We all understand that much of who we are comes from the expression of our genes that we inherited from our families of origin. The color of our eyes, our height, the texture of our hair—we can see these patterns develop and mix across generations in ways that are obvious and undeniable. They are remarked on even when they depart from the pattern. When the daughter of a 5'6" man and a 5'2" woman grows to be 6' tall, it's worth remarking on—where did she come from? If you look back, usually you can find some towering great aunt or maternal cousin who also stood head and shoulders above her siblings. "Oh," we say, "it must have skipped a generation."

But of course, it didn't really "skip" a generation. It just lay dormant and unexpressed in one generation. These are obvious physical characteristics, but what we inherit from our parents and grandparents is more than skin deep.

Many people have the misconception that our genetic state is static. We are born with half of our chromosomes from our mother and half from our father, and that combination determines our appearance, our susceptibility to disease and disorder, our blood type, and other features. But what many people are missing from their understanding of genetics is that environments and behaviors can change how your genes work and how they are expressed in your body well beyond the moment of conception. Epigenetics refers to the influence of environmental factors on genetic expression and explores how these genetic expressions can also be inherited from generation to generation.

Stress caused by illness, malnutrition, and trauma can influence the production of proteins in your body on the cellular and genetic levels. These proteins are fundamental components of all your body's complex systems, including your nervous system and brain.

Take diabetes, for example. Many of us have the genetic predisposition for diabetes in our inherited genetic code, and it might never "wake up" and cause an active presentation of the disease. Environmental factors like stress, poor nutrition, unhealthy lifestyle, or lack of prenatal care can epigenetically change the expression of genes in such a way that wakes up that predisposition for diabetes and makes it much more likely that the next generation struggles with the disease in a way that previous generations may not have.

We can understand that neurological issues are exacerbated by environmental factors, but it's also important to recognize that these, too, can be passed along. SUD is one of these disorders that might be heightened by genetic history. There are many reasons why someone may use substances to solve any number of internal problems. Some common ones include social anxiety, where consuming a substance can calm our nerves by offering a bit of ease. Others can be uncomfortable in their bodies and need to alter the way they feel physically to be comfortable being with others. Some may feel simply bored and need a shift in perspective or excitement to feel like they're engaging with the community. Others may experience chronic physical pain. Nothing on this list is something that a person wouldn't naturally want to fix—to find any solution for— even if it's a temporary one.

While the exact nature of the brain chemistry varies and continues to be studied, repeated use of substances creates a cyclical reward path in the brain, which changes the neurochemical makeup of the individual over time, including epigenetic changes. This capacity can be heightened in the next generation, increasing the likelihood that substance use may escalate into a disorder.

Of course, this is not a matter of one-to-one cause and effect; it's a part of the greater picture we can use to help develop our understanding and self-compassion. It's also important to understand because, unlike the genome, epigenetic changes can be reversed.

In my support of families, I have seen how epigenetic understanding of our past can help empower us to make changes for the future. A family that I worked with experienced the loss of a child when their son was very young. The traumatic loss understandably affected the parents' ability to engage in their lives for quite a while and forever changed the way they parented their other children. The parents immersed themselves in their professions. Their young son experienced confusion and felt a lack of love and even abandonment.

As he grew up, he began to struggle with unhealthy relationships and ultimately turned to substance use to fill the void he felt as a child. He carried a lot of anger, and the family worked hard to understand that their behaviors during a very impactful time in their son's life had caused feelings of detachment, abandonment, and loss. As responsible as he was for the pain caused by his current actions, he was perpetuating that because he didn't know any other way to find connection but through unhealthy attachments to women and substances.

It was not an easy thing to grapple with for the family, but stepping back and looking at the bigger picture gave them the space they needed to find the strength to change. They could work together with their son to try to stop the cycle of disconnection and suffering.

⌒⌒

One tool that can be helpful for families to explore how generational patterns may be affecting their current lives is called a genogram. Superficially, a genogram resembles a family tree, but it can contain much more information than simple lineage and marriage history. Using various symbols and color-coding, a genogram can also depict instances of certain genetically passed disorders like heart disease, dementia, diabetes, major mental health disorders, and even addictions. This can visually reveal these patterns through generations. By using a genogram, we can also consider the different timelines and contexts and how previous generations may have coped (or tried to cope) with these patterns. This allows us to see which patterns—both behavioral and genetic —may have been passed down to us.

In addition to the traditional branches of a family tree, genograms can also employ symbols to show emotional and interpersonal relationships. If a relationship between a child and parent or between parents of children is abusive or violent, this can be marked with a red, jagged line. If there is a close bond of friendship between cousins, step-siblings, or family-in-law, this can be shown through dotted green lines. Genograms can also show losses like miscarriages, childhood deaths, and even breaks in communication between family members. Examining these charts can reveal potential connections between traumatic events and inherited traits.

A genogram of three to five generations can show some amazing patterns that might illuminate dynamics within the contemporary generation. For a simple example, a genogram may reveal that four generations back, a mother and father experienced malnutrition and food insecurity during *An Gorta Mór*, also known as Ireland's Great Hunger or Potato Famine. While they crossed the Atlantic by "coffin ship," fear and strife defining their existence, their epigenetic expression was profoundly affected. This was passed to their children, the first generation born in America. This subsequent generation may have greater issues with heart disease, stroke, and coping through substance use.

Another generation down the line brings us to the Great Depression, which marks another generation with periods of high stress and poor nutrition. The contemporary descendants of this family line may continue to feel the effects of these centuries-old periods of trauma and desperation through higher rates of diabetes and heart ailments, and they also may experience disordered relationships with food through both genetic expression and inherited behaviors built up around those remembered periods of extreme food insecurity and stress.

Taking a broader look at these patterns does not undo the pattern of stress and trauma, but understanding them can lead to both empathy for family members and a greater capacity for self-compassion. This knowledge helps contemporary generations make informed decisions about their health and behaviors.

Some patterns revealed in genograms can show how substance use travels through generations, but it can reveal other patterns as well. Some of these patterns reflect cultural influences and changes over time. The personal identity of being a caregiver, for example, has often been passed down through generations of women. For the contemporary woman's great-great-grandmother, acting as caregiver to her family was likely not only central to her identity but one of the limited options for survival and security.

Emotional enmeshment—an excessive emotional involvement in another, leading to a blurring or lack of personal autonomy—may have served a survival purpose for the women of these previous generations. When their security was entirely dependent on their husbands or fathers and their futures were secured by their sons, it made sense that these women developed a strong sensitivity to their men's emotional state and developed coping mechanisms that included managing their family's emotional state. This pattern of emotional enmeshment entangled with an identity of caregiving can be passed along, and these patterns no longer serve a survival purpose. In working with families, I have seen this pattern emerge. Just as substance use is passed through generations, so are emotionally enmeshed attachment styles.

Understanding these patterns is one way of stepping back and reflecting on your behaviors and actions in a broader scope. This process is not about finding blame or pushing off the responsibility of how you show up in the world. It can be an empowering act because when you see and understand the pattern, you can *change* the pattern.

You and every member of your family have a place within the broader pattern. If part of that pattern is not working, it will be expressed in different ways in different individuals, whether it is through substance use or some other coping mechanism.

In studying my family's genogram, I discovered two significant patterns: One was a history of mental illness that presented in various ways, and the other was a habit of keeping secrets to protect ourselves and others. To start to heal and do better, I had to find a way to step out of the pattern as much as I could.

There's much still to be learned in the field of epigenetics. I'm hopeful that more therapies will be developed—both mental and physical—to holistically account for these epigenetic influences and their role in SUD.

For us, as the families of people in an immediate and continuing struggle with SUD, epigenetics has a more immediate role. Epigenetics can teach us that there is a greater context to these issues and remind us that some of the influences we're seeing are buried deep in our very being. To understand this is not to relinquish any of our responsibility. Things that aren't working are still ours to own and address. But we can't address the problem if we treat it as an isolated issue—a blemish on otherwise unmarked skin —that can simply be excised.

Trying to cover it up or force it away is often a perpetuation of family coping mechanisms that have not worked for generations. Previous generations typically had fewer choices and did what they could manage at the time, so assigning blame or finding root causes is not our goal when we examine family patterns.

By understanding that this problem is the current expression of a pattern, we can find a greater feeling of empathy for our people and ourselves, and we can empower ourselves to break free from that pattern and model it differently for future generations.

When you invite your person into this healing process, you can help them recognize the problem as well. This is a fundamental change in communication and connection because you are no longer focusing on the behavior or telling them that they are the problem and they must change. We are modeling to them that something is not working for us, but *together* we can fix it. We are saying that something is not working, and it is being expressed in one way in you and other ways in us. We're going to do the work to change this and break the pattern the best we can.

We'd love for you to join us.

PART TWO

PSYCHOEDUCATION

CHAPTER 5

YOUR BRAIN IN SURVIVAL MODE

OUR BRAINS ARE, first and foremost, geared to ensure our survival. When we believe that survival is under threat, thoughts of reasonable actions or carefully weighed choices or potential consequences go out the window. If you've ever felt that sudden rush of fear or shock that triggers a fight-or-flight response, even for a fleeting moment, you can understand that your next few actions can easily be out of character for you.

If the fear is prolonged, the out-of-character behavior will be too.

I used to compete in triathlons. The beginning of a triathlon can be fairly brutal and sometimes dangerous, with dozens up to hundreds of people running to get into the water and get their swimming rhythm established as quickly as possible. The beginning can be very crowded as the athletes strive for the best possible position in the water. The chill of water itself can be a shock to the senses as you try to focus on keeping your muscles moving. Once, just as I was getting fully into the deeper water and trying to find some room to swim, I felt a hand hit my ankle—and then wrap around it.

The woman behind me pulled me down into the water, and I felt her swim up and over me. In that moment, I was terrified. There was water up my nose, and I hadn't taken a good enough breath to be submerged the way I was. The lake water was opaque around me, and I couldn't see. I felt the woman swim over me, blocking me from the surface and pushing me deeper. I felt the water around me churn as other swimmers kicked around me. They couldn't see me, and soon, I was being beaten up by strong legs kicking to find their thrust in the water.

My survival brain was screaming at me that I couldn't breathe. I was underwater and no longer felt in control. Drowning didn't just feel like a possibility; it was something imminently happening. Everything around me felt like a deadly enemy. I flailed my arms to make it back to the surface as fast as possible.

If anything—anyone—had been still in my way, still between me and the surface, I know I would have punched, clawed, kicked, or pushed them with everything I had. I would have grabbed an arm or leg and pulled someone down just as the woman had pulled me down. At that moment, those actions would have made complete sense to me.

None of that is in my nature, but what is in your nature feels very different when you think you're drowning. When your lungs have little air and you're surrounded by dark waters, that survival mechanism kicks in, and nothing else matters other than securing your next breath—you will do what it takes to get it.

I got back to the surface, of course, and after a few seconds of regaining my bearings and breath, I got back into my swimming rhythm. I added quite a bit of distance to my swim by taking the time to go out into the open water to separate myself from the others. I didn't want to experience that again. I was back in control and could make decisions again, but I still remembered what it felt like to be under. I still remember it now.

Someone in the midst of active addiction is always underwater.

The survival part of the brain is in the limbic system. It's the deep, primal part of the brain, with the amygdala, thalamus, and the cingulate gyrus. The limbic system also includes structures such as the nucleus accumbens and the ventral tegmental area (VTA), which are key components of the brain's reward pathway. When a person engages in a pleasurable activity, such as eating, socializing, or drinking alcohol and taking drugs, these areas release dopamine, a neurotransmitter associated with pleasure and reward. This intense dopamine surge creates a strong sense of euphoria and pleasure.

The limbic system is where our emotions live, the fear and pleasure responses, autonomic functions like thirst and hunger, and the hardwiring of core, long-term memories. It's where addiction lives and takes root. The pleasure center and the survival response center are intertwined in this section of the brain, and they affect each other.

Substance use often starts in response to emotional discomfort as a way to feel good—or even just a little bit better—in the moment. The discomfort itself could stem from what we might call "Big T Trauma," like injurious accidents, loss from natural disasters, violence, illness, or the sudden loss of a loved one or caregiver. Not everyone who develops SUD has one of these big-T sources of pain. However, there are also many little-t trauma sources, like bullying; shame; losses of relationships through moving, divorce, or life changes; feelings of isolation or insecurity in childhood; loss of a job or other financial stress; and memories of humiliation or failure.

Substance use works temporarily to ease this discomfort and replace it with positive feelings. Depending on the substance and circumstances, the person may be looking to lose weight, alleviate boredom or social anxiety, fall asleep more easily, or simulate a feeling of sharp focus or concentration. When the substance feels effective for that purpose, the behavior is reinforced. The person may feel excited and euphoric, more socially connected, at ease or relaxed, productive, or simply not in emotional or physical pain. The feedback in the brain from the substance use is that it *worked*.

When a behavior feels like it works, the brain reinforces it by calling for the behavior again. And again. And again.

The behavior of seeking the substance is continually reinforced, so it always makes sense to the person using substances. It continues to make sense to them even as they get more and more extreme in seeking out substances. In this way, SUD enters through the pleasure center like a virus can come into the body through the lungs.

The memories formed during these heightened pleasure states are embedded into the hippocampus, such that environmental cues trigger the intense cravings and compulsive drug-seeking behavior that can grow more intense over time and lead to increasingly dangerous behaviors. The use of substances began to fulfill a need —one that, on the surface, was completely understandable—but after repeated use, the original need is completely overshadowed by the new constant need for the substance itself.

The chemistry of addiction is complicated and varies somewhat by the type of substances used. With stimulants like cocaine or methamphetamine, the levels of dopamine are briefly maxed out, and the natural reuptake and release is blocked and disrupted. Soon, it seems to the person that to feel capable of pleasure at all, they must continue using the drug. Depressants like alcohol and benzodiazepines (benzos) calm neural activity and reduce the immediate sensations of stress. Over time, they take over the brain's ability to self-regulate, causing elevated levels of stress and pain during any period of sobriety. Opioids bind to opioid receptors in the brain, mimicking the effects of endorphins, relieving pain, and causing euphoria.

Whatever the variation of chemical that is being used, the basic process is the same. Through repeated use, the substance will hijack the whole limbic system until it's no longer about scratching an itch, easing pain, or engaging the pleasure center. Eventually, the brain feels that the substance is absolutely essential to its continued function.

After a longer period of repeated use, the purpose of using substances or drinking is no longer to feel good but to stop feeling sick. The sickness and physical and emotional pain that become associated with the need for the substance become tied up with the need to eat, breathe, hydrate, and sleep. It becomes such an essential need that the person may choose the substance over food, sleeping, or safety. It becomes hardwired to the extent that, at times, they feel they will die without that substance.

For the person living through that experience, that fear couldn't be more real. The brain thinks, "I need this to survive," and the message is just as present and immediate as if they were being held underwater. When that level of fear activates, the person would fight, kick, or steal to get the substance they use, just as they would in the face of the threat of violent death. They would do things completely outside their normal character because the primal part of the brain is affected *that* drastically by long-term substance use.

With some substances in high-frequency use, suddenly stopping can be dangerous and even fatal, as with alcohol or benzodiazepines. Other drugs, like most opioids, should be monitored by professionals but, in most cases, will not be dangerous, only extremely uncomfortable and even physically painful.

For those of us on the outside of the experience of addiction, that prospect is terrifying to think about. It is baffling to us why someone would take such a risk. Even more baffling is why they would compile risk on risk to keep seeking the substance. From our perspective, it makes no sense. That's why so many well-meaning family members have conversation after conversation, trying to explain the dangers and appeal to their person's sense of reason. People experiencing SUD often already know these dangers. If the solution were as simple as sharing information, recovery would be much more straightforward. Very few people can detox from opioids without help because the sensation of need is that powerful. Going without feels like dying, like being held underwater, like the worst kind of sickness. The need to make that feeling stop is overpowering. It's primal.

When we witness someone we love making choices that we cannot fathom, it's easy to feel like the person is totally lost or changed. So often, I hear families talk about their loved ones in the past tense and about their current actions and behavior as if they are being committed by some malevolent stranger who has taken their place. Families are hurt and confused when their loved ones lie to them, steal from them, yell at them, or try any manipulation they can think of for money or whatever else they need to continue their substance use. Someone being held under the waters of SUD will say whatever they need to in order to get what they feel they need, no matter how much it might hurt you. They may become unrecognizable in that behavior. In a way, they *are* a stranger because when you communicate with someone deep in SUD, you are no longer communicating with your person but with the disorder.

Picture your person in a room. They are sitting in a corner, desperate, sad, and broken. There is another being in that room. That second being is impulsive and irrational. That being thinks it's protecting your person while they retreat into the corner. It guards the door. It calls the shots.

This being is their addiction. When you are at the door, trying to reason with them, your message is not getting to the person you love because it is deflected by the addiction. All the fight-or-flight mechanisms of survival have become re-centered around the need for the substance. Their addiction is in a constant state of need and desperation.

When you feel like you've lost your person to another unrecognizable person who is showing up to the door, remember your person is still there in the corner, unable to hear your messages. Separate from their difficult behavior, they are still the same person you love and want to repair a connection with. It is for that person that we need to hold space for empathy and understanding.

The more we can understand the complexities of SUD, the more we can compassionately interpret their behavior. Before you can step in and be effective in helping them, we need to learn how to understand their behavior and the reasons—logical to us or not— behind their choices. Every individual is different, so there is no script to learn or specific pattern of moves to identify. When you have more understanding of the nature of the disease, you can think about their behavior differently and shift your family's focus from changing the behavior to connecting with the person. Instead of focusing on how the behavior looks on the outside, you can focus on why it makes sense to them.

∿

The neurochemistry behind behavior is powerful, and there is still a lot to learn and understand. In truth, science has just scratched the surface of how social, emotional, and cultural influences work together with the chemistry, biology, and psychology in the brain. As important as it is to have clarity about how much brain chemistry is affecting the behavior of our person, it is equally important to remember that we, too, have brains with chemical and neurological pathways that deeply affect our behavior and our experience of the world.

In chapter three, I referenced the pause, the space between stimulus and response in which the freedom and responsibility to make choices exists. Stimuli come from the environment, but they also come from within our brains. For instance, hunger and thirst both originate in the limbic system of the brain. They are simple chemical triggers that tell us to seek out food and drink. They are deeply linked to both our basic survival and our health and well- being, and the brain does its best to regularly use these triggers to maintain positive homeostasis in the body with all that it needs to function well. These chemical impulses can also be muddied by other things—smells, boredom, anxiety, and memories of pleasure can generate that same sensation of hunger.

These impulses can be harder to recognize as stimuli because they are intricately a part of us, coming from within. However, we can still make use of the pause. Feeling hungry but choosing to wait forty-five minutes to eat because of context or convenience doesn't take anything like the kind of will and effort that overcoming stronger and deeper impulses does, but the *pause* makes both choices equally possible.

Of all of the ways that outside stimuli can affect our brain chemistry, there is none that can wholly manufacture a feeling or experience in the brain that doesn't exist there in some form already. Pleasure, fear, and the need for touch or love are all existing pathways in our brains. Substance use is just one way those pathways are deepened and altered. Pathways in the mind can be eroded into ditches, then trenches, then deep fissures. What starts as a way to trigger ease and pleasure can develop into a belief that their substance is the only thing that can secure survival. The way out gets harder to reach as the recurring behavior becomes more ingrained over time, but it's always there.

Substance use may start out as a response to a feeling similar to hunger. But we have to remember that as the use is repeated and deepens into a disorder, the feeling morphs. It's no longer the feeling of hunger but much closer to the need *not to starve*. Remembering this helps us understand what our person is experiencing with a bit more clarity.

With that understanding in place, we can also consider how our own chemistry is affecting our behavior. Repeated fear and stress can create chemical ruts in our minds that make us reach for the wrong tools to cope, such as anger, control, or self-sacrifice.

When we react in these ways, we are also provided with a neurological reward, reinforcing that behavior despite its ineffectiveness in achieving what we actually want. In this way, like our loved and struggling person, we have our own neurological pattern to disrupt.

We are *all* more than the sum of the electrical impulses in our gray matter, but those structures are very much a part of who we are. To recover, both for ourselves and our person, we have to consider the whole person, including all the electrochemical impulses that influence our behavior, for better and for worse.

I don't know why that swimmer in the triathlon pulled me under, but I know I would have done the same to her or someone else if it was what it took to get me out from under that water. Perhaps, somewhere in the chaotic churn of water behind me, she had also lost connection to the surface and her feeling of control. Pulling me under may have made complete sense to her at the time.

Finding room for understanding does not mean agreeing with hurtful behavior. There is never a point where we stop being responsible for our actions and their consequences. However, in engaging with each other, we can endeavor to understand when actions are made out of a sense of desperation. The survival instinct is the most powerful impulse of the brain, the central drive that all other impulses serve. When it is hijacked, it takes enormous work and strength to overcome that feeling and act differently. When it is hijacked, it is difficult to feel anything else.

For a person with SUD, the neurochemical pathways that have been altered by the substance use can be remapped with time and healing. Our own neurological ruts can also be remapped to serve us better. Stepping into the work of remapping our reactions to be more responsive can model the way for our person. To be of help to them, we must understand our own patterns first.

CHAPTER 6

HARM REDUCTION VERSUS ABSORBING HARM

SAVING someone's life doesn't always look like you'd expect.

For example, one young man—whose drug of choice was fentanyl—entered treatment. Shortly after, he called his family and simply told them he wasn't ready to quit yet. Leaving treatment to continue his use left him experiencing homelessness, as his behavior was not safe for this family to be close to. He knew the consequences, and for a period of time, he chose it. To say this was a scary situation is a huge understatement—this is a nightmare scenario for parents.

It's easy to imagine a fantasy of swooping into action to save the day, like something from a movie—you comb the city for your child, track them down, and throw them into the car. Once they're contained, you finally say all the right words in the right order, and miraculously, they see the light. Everything suddenly makes sense to them. You heroically drive them back to treatment, but this time, you know it will stick. You save their life, whether they like it or not, and believe the gratitude will come later when it's finally behind you and you can all rest easy.

But recovery never works without active participation from the person in treatment. There are no magic right words to say in a magic right order. That's why this story is a fantasy.

That's not what the parents of this young man did.

They had anticipated the struggles would continue and had intentional, thought-through boundaries in place, and those boundaries meant they would not try to swoop in to save the day. They provided their son with a cell phone so they could stay connected, but they didn't provide a data plan, requiring him to be near a public place in order to connect. They knew that being in public meant he could be seen by others and that, in times of acute distress, public places provide the potential for faster help and medical attention if needed. Of course, when they could speak with their son, they used that time to listen to him and left the solutions out of the words they spoke. He knew where they stood; what they would support was his recovery. But still, he wasn't ready. He couldn't stop, and he didn't want to—yet.

Arguing wouldn't have been effective, and it would have strained the relationship even further, so they didn't argue. Instead, they asked him a hard question.

"Can we help you not die?"

It's hard to imagine saying those words to someone you love. It's much easier to imagine the save-the-day scenario of tracking them down and throwing them over your shoulder, hauling them off to somewhere you can hold them until they're better.

It hurts to voice this question because it acknowledges the very real potential result of your person's choices.

Thankfully, his answer was yes, I will take that help. He didn't want to die.

So they connected him with harm reduction resources. The harm reduction strategies for fentanyl are extensive because of the nature of the drug, and in this case, they included sterile needles and a support person to sit with him with Narcan as he used.

It may seem strange to refer to this type of support as "safety measures," but that's exactly what they are. During this relapse, he was unhoused for six weeks. There is no telling what could have happened without those measures in place. The "saving the day" fantasy wouldn't have worked—that has been proven time and time again. But these measures may well have been the only thing that kept him alive.

After those six weeks, he called his family. He was ready. He went into detox in the early hours of the next morning, and, as of this writing, he is living a life in recovery and has been for years.

It was an unimaginable scenario, but in the end, it was evidence of what can happen when families become a part of harm-reduction strategies.

There are many misconceptions regarding harm reduction when it comes to SUD. But in other areas of life, you probably use harm-reduction strategies regularly. Applying sunscreen when we go outdoors for extended periods and wearing a helmet while biking are acts of harm reduction. Like many actions we regularly take, spending too much time in the sun and riding a bike both carry the possibility of harm. Using these harm-reducing strategies simply makes the harm less likely or less severe. Most often, we use harm-reduction strategies when we intend to do a potentially harmful activity regardless of its potential dangers. The same is true of harm-reduction practices in the context of combating the harms of drug or alcohol use.

Anyone who has made use of or volunteered to be a designated driver while drinking has participated in harm-reduction practices surrounding substance use, but of course, this strategy doesn't usually provoke controversy. Those who oppose harm-reduction practices are usually reacting to cases where the strategy includes needle exchanges, counteractive substances like Narcan, and safe-use spaces. Many feel that these provisions are equivalent to condoning the behavior.

Often, the term "enabling"—which is frequently misused and even weaponized in policies surrounding SUD treatment—is applied to harm-reduction strategies, but the two concepts are fundamentally different. "Enabling" involves actions that inadvertently support or empower destructive behaviors, shielding individuals from the consequences of their actions. Harm reduction is not about condoning the behavior, nor is it about "giving in" to the nature of substance use by providing limitless amounts of the substance.

In a clinical context, harm reduction is a mainstream approach to managing substance use until a person is ready to take further action in their recovery. It is compassionate and pragmatic, and it acknowledges both the harsh realities of substance use and the importance of honoring your person's autonomy. The primary goal is first to reduce harm, but the approach also seeks to build bridges to healing and impactful connections to those affected by SUD.

As a matter of public policy, harm reduction has its roots in the early 1980s. In the midst of the rapidly growing HIV/AIDS crisis, it was discovered that needle sharing and intravenous drug use were a major path of the disease's spread. Needle Exchange Programs (NEPs) were developed to help combat this branch of the problem and curb the spread. The first program was arranged in Amsterdam in 1983, and evidence showed that it had a significant impact on transmission rates. And it did *not* increase the use of intravenous drugs, as some feared it would. The United States adopted the practice in the late 1980s, and though it was a highly controversial program, evidence showed it had enormous benefits.

Not only did NEPs help curb the spread of HIV and other blood-borne diseases like hepatitis, but they also provided people who used IV drugs with a new avenue to seek other and more significant forms of treatment. NEPs were designed to be non-stigmatizing because they had to be attractive to be effective and reach people where they were. As people engaged with the services from NEPs, they also had additional access to information for other potential services in a judgment-free and inviting environment. Evidence showed that NEPs also increased access to and use of mental health services, detox, and SUD treatment programs.

The reason we want to intervene in someone's substance use is not the substance itself but the *harm* the substance can and will cause physically, psychologically, and socially. When we see what that substance can do to our person, we naturally grow to focus on and hate the substance itself. It's a very human response. This perspective can make harm-reduction practices feel like a step in the wrong direction; giving a sterile needle to someone can feel like giving them drugs.

But this may be a misplaced emotional trigger. To make the best, informed, and reasonable choices regarding what strategies and avenues we support, we have to remember that it is the *harm* that poses the danger. NEPs do not endorse intravenous drug use, nor do they create a culture where it's fine "in moderation." They simply acknowledge that, in the range of dangerous behaviors, intravenous use with a sterile needle is safer than use with one that can carry disease. If that is the only step towards a healthier life that is available for a person on that day, then it's one worth taking.

This is the same strategy represented by Narcan. Just as needle exchanges were developed in response to the existing AIDS crisis, Narcan (naloxone, generically) was developed to reverse opioid overdoses.

Naloxone was first synthesized in the 1960s by Dr. Jack Fishman and Dr. Solomon Snyder. An opioid overdose can be lethal when it causes severe respiratory depression, which means the person's breathing slows down significantly or stops altogether. Opioids depress the central nervous system, and when taken in high doses, they can overwhelm the body's ability to maintain normal respiratory function. This lack of oxygen can result in brain damage or death if not promptly treated.

Narcan works by displacing opioids that are causing life-threatening respiratory depression. This rapid reversal restores normal breathing, often within minutes, providing a critical window for further medical intervention. Narcan has evolved into a widely accessible and easy-to-administer form, including nasal spray versions that require no medical training to use.

The mechanics of an opioid overdose existed for centuries before the countermeasure was researched and developed. The scary potential for overdose itself was not enough to deter its use across both medical and recreational contexts, so Narcan was developed in order to *keep people breathing*. The purpose of Narcan is not to pave the way for continued opioid use; it is to preserve life.

Embracing harm-reduction strategies can also be beneficial for substance use not associated with needles or opioids. Broadly speaking, it is a mindset focused on doing what we can with compassion and understanding. When professionally implemented, harm reduction is about extending life and avoiding permanent physical damage, which provides *more* opportunity for your person to choose to stop using substances, not less.

Before introducing harm reduction as a potential strategy for your person and your family, it's important to become informed of the options and, whenever possible, use professional guidance and advice. From the position of family members, harm reduction is about providing information and resources, rather than opinions and judgment, to support your person as they choose safer behaviors. Open, honest, and non-judgmental conversations with your loved one are the first step. Listen to their experiences and concerns without imposing your will. Create a safe space for dialogue so you can understand their unique journey and needs. You'll only be able to offer alternative solutions once connection and predictable communication are established.

Depending on your circumstances and the substance involved, you can encourage safety measures like using sterile needles, fentanyl test strips, and Narcan to reverse overdoses. Encourage your loved one to avoid using substances alone and to have a friend present when they do. This can help mitigate the risk of overdose or other dangerous situations. Asking the question "Do you ensure your safety by having someone with you and carrying Narcan?" demonstrates that you care about their life first and foremost and encourages them to make the safest choices available to them in their behavior.

Appropriate harm reduction practices do not ask you as the family member to actively participate in the process. In fact, families can also use harm-reduction strategies for themselves since forming and keeping boundaries allows us to ensure our safety and well-being, which is crucial in all stages of recovery, theirs and ours.

For instance, harm-reduction strategies do *not* require you to make your home a "safe site" for your person to use. Encouraging them to have someone with them in a clean and safe space does not mean that *you* should sit with them while in active use in your home. Providing that for them directly could further entangle your relationship. Sacrificing your security—whether it is financial, emotional, or your physical home—may not reduce the overall harm but merely shift it around.

Other measures, like simply having Narcan on hand, do not require you to absorb risk or break your necessary boundaries but may be used to save your person's life. Each circumstance is different. It can be difficult to support your person separately from their behavior, especially when the two have become entangled, so the more you can learn about the options available, the better you can support them.

Learn about the specific substance your loved one is struggling with. Understanding its effects, risks, and available resources can help you provide better support and specific actions that your person may actually be able to take. The Substance Abuse and Mental Health Services Administration (SAMHSA) offers a national helpline and resources for finding local treatment and harm reduction services, and the National Harm Reduction Coalition website is a source for up-to-date information on practices and available strategies.

Harm-reduction strategies do not start with family members engaging in the services directly but with conversations and sharing information with your person so they can have the option to choose safer behaviors even if they aren't ready to stop the behavior altogether. In many ways, keeping this in mind helps maintain sensible boundaries and that delicate balance between support and accountability. The mindset of harm reduction strategies is rooted in autonomy and empowerment, so your person needs to make the active choice to engage with the practices.

When our son was in active addiction, my husband and I did everything we could to both pull him back and keep him safe. We knew that what he was doing was more than dangerous; it was potentially deadly. We also wanted to be there to catch him if he lost control. He's our son, and we wanted to protect him from everything we possibly could.

Thinking about that time, my husband describes us as though we were watching him run back and forth across a tightrope. The tightrope was far, far above our heads, and there was no net. In our fear for him, we ran along the ground, holding a small exercise trampoline between us—a farce of safety and the image of futility. We exhausted ourselves holding on to this metaphorical trampoline. For years, we expended feverish energy trying to take back our son's responsibility for his life.

Our behaviors communicated two things that we never even considered. First, our actions told him that he wasn't capable without us. And second, they communicated that he would always be okay because we were there to catch him if he fell.

Neither of those things was true.

Fear does not prevent someone from dying.

He was far too high on that tightrope. If he had fallen, there was nothing our toy of a trampoline could do. Secondly, all the running exhausted us, hurt us, and cost us our health and well-being.

Harm reduction is *not* absorbing harm. Reducing harm cannot mean taking harm on yourself. Adopting the risks and burdens of substance use or deflecting the consequences of the behavior doesn't take the harm away—it just takes the harm on yourself while providing no additional safety to your person.

Our fear led us to feel that our son wasn't capable of things without us, but that was just as false as the veneer of a safety net that we were trying to provide.

Many families who are supporting a family member with SUD, over the course of years, become significantly financially entangled with them, taking on more and more of the bills. The instinct to do this stems from the story that they never *have* done things without help, so they *cannot* do things without help. They are not adequately taking care of themselves, and loving family members step in to take up the slack. They may even pay off drug debts, hoping that if they can prevent those consequences long enough, then there will be a wake-up call before the harm and damage become too much to deflect.

This is not harm reduction. In fact, it extends harm and spreads it further into the future and throughout the family. It is absorbing harm. Paying their rent or mortgage, paying for their food delivery, or paying to fix their car will not heal their brain and take away the emotional pain that is at the root of their substance use.

That is not to say that all financial support is bad. Every situation is different, and you will have to account for both your person's circumstances and your personal and family values. The kinds of support you give should be carefully examined and considered. Ask yourself whether your actions are empowering them or easing your own discomfort. Are you just running around with an exercise trampoline?

I often invite families to ask themselves to what degree—what percentage—they believe in their person's ability to achieve independence. If you are paying someone's mortgage, is it because they will become homeless if you don't, or is it that *you're afraid* that they will? If you're paying for food delivery, would they really starve without it? Is your support providing safety and a potential path to health and support, or is it providing comfort and ease for you and perpetuating the story that everything is ok for them?

The fact that your person is not currently taking care of themselves doesn't necessarily mean that they can't. If you make changes to that comfort and ease you are providing, there may be real and measurable consequences for them, often starting with financial trouble. These consequences actually provide an opportunity for clarity. If you are carrying burdens that belong to your person, neither you nor they have data about what will happen when and if you put them down. That data is needed for everyone to have clarity on the nature and the scope of the problem. When faced with the reality that they cannot continue independently the way they have been, many people will find the motivation to look for ways to change the status quo.

The purpose of harm reduction is *not* to support every part of a person's life while they are in active addiction. It may feel better—more logical—to give someone money for food or housing than it does to provide clean needles, Narcan, or the address of a safe-use site. Many people feel like providing these safety measures gives "permission" for their person to continue using.

But your person doesn't need your permission. They have already given themselves permission. The food deliveries and secure housing just allow them to continue to put their energy into maintaining their active addiction and feeding the increasingly demanding need in their brain.

Absorbing the burden of their financial, housing, and food security does not honor their autonomy, and it may not get them any closer to recovery. But while it may feel counter-intuitive, providing some safety measures during active addiction can help ensure they make it to the day that they're ready for change.

No one can recover if they're dead.

The more you understand about the available tools and practices, the more you can provide the mental health support your person needs and give them options that can lessen the harm their substance use brings without absorbing that harm on their behalf.

CHAPTER 7

THE PAUSE

"STOP" and "think" are words most of us hear from a young age. This advice is one of those fundamental things children must learn in order to avoid hurt. When we see a young child acting impulsively—running toward something they want or throwing something they don't—the potential consequences are obvious to us. That lesson of "stop and think" is shared repeatedly and with urgency throughout childhood. Look both ways before crossing the street. Think before you speak. Look around you for solutions before you react. The message is reinforced in all kinds of ways.

Given that this is one of the most elementary lessons we learn in early life, it can seem painfully oversimplified to us once we reach adulthood. Surely, we all know how to stop and think by now. So why is it so hard to do when the rubber meets the road?

As children, our impulses are simple, and the potential hurt is equally one-dimensional. We learn to control these simple impulses as an automatic process of growing up. But as we grow up, our impulses grow more complicated. The potential outcomes are also more complex and difficult to predict or account for. Our desires and needs contradict and pull us in opposite directions. When this happens, more than ever, we need to stop and think before we take actions that will have myriad impacts on those around us, for better or for worse.

Most of us don't actually struggle with the "think" part. Our brains are constant machines, going and going and imagining scenarios and outcomes and reaching for solutions. Our minds can be like beehives, a million thoughts working together, or sometimes at cross-purposes.

The stopping part is more difficult.

In previous chapters, I have talked about the important concept of the pause. We can take advantage of that space between stimulus and response to make choices. In that space, there is freedom to make intentional choices that represent your values and beliefs.

But using that space requires that we stop there and exist in it for a time. We have to actively pull ourselves to a halt so that we can really see with clarity what our true choices are and how previous choices have brought us to this moment. Sometimes, it's easier said than done.

To give ourselves a moment to stop and think, we need something to hold on to. That something is our connection to our person, understood through a lens of our values and our love for them.

Your love is how you feel for your person, but your connection is a two-way street. Connection is how you express love in a way that can be felt by them. When you can stop reacting to your person's behavior and sit in the pause, responding in a way that your love can be received, connection happens. Stopping the cycle of your reaction sometimes means stopping action altogether, at least for a time. Stillness is hard, even for short periods of time, when it feels like we are in crisis. When we believe we are in crisis, that belief tends to overpower and shut out all else, including our ability to stop and think.

Taking a pause can feel inactive, particularly when our brain is telling us to act. But pausing is not doing nothing; it's actually part of taking the hard-easy path. When we take a pause and disrupt our instincts to constantly react, we give ourselves the room to start that hard work that will make future actions easier and more effective.

To change our circumstances, especially patterns of behavior that we get stuck in, we have to stop and think. When we do, we can find the quiet we need to get clarity.

I worked with a mother whose son had spiraled for many years as he regularly used drugs. For years, she was doing everything she could to get him to stop, constantly communicating the dangers to her son in hopes she could persuade him to stop. But her pleas were always met with unyielding resistance and resentment from him.

She sent him statistics and articles about the irreparable damage of the drug he was using. He asked her to stop, he begged her to stop, and he stopped answering her calls and texts. She sent him social media shorts and posts from people in recovery and doctors on the harms of using. He responded, *Mom, stop.*

In each conversation, she begged him to tell her what she could do to make him stop and seek recovery. He just told her to stop. This cycle continued for years, this back and forth that never moved the needle.

Finally, she started the work of Parallel Recovery. She stopped to think about what she could do differently to focus on healing herself and her pain. She realized that she had never really heard him say it.

Stop.

She looked back at the dozens of messages and threads, and she realized that she had been unable to hear him before. Her pain was too loud. Her *need* for him to be better—because it would allow *her* to feel better—drowned out his pleas.

Son, I need you to stop.

Mom, I need you to stop.

When she was finally able to look back at their communication patterns, she found a new clarity. The cycle of "stops" was only driving both of their pain and straining their connection to each other.

This is not to say she had to switch to condoning his behavior or accepting his excuses or justifications for his behavior. Instead of telling him about the irreversible damage he was causing to his body and mind, she told him that she was sorry he was hurting. When he tried to tell her that his use wasn't really a problem—when he tried to justify his "safe usage"—she learned to close the subject. She held firm to her boundary of no longer talking about his behavior of drug use.

But she knew that insisting there was no safe usage and loading him with more and more information about the harms of his drug use was not serving either of them. It couldn't be her role in the relationship anymore. The information was there, and he knew it. She didn't need to share more. And she didn't need to listen to his justifications for using or engage him in conversations late at night when he was high.

She had desperately wanted to help him. She just didn't realize that the best way to accomplish that goal was to help herself first. In getting the support she needed, she gave herself the space to move toward healing and model what "stopping and thinking" could look like for her son.

A pause is the last thing a panicked brain wants to take.

You might even now be feeling, *but no... I can't... but, but, but...*

It's not easy. It's the hard part of the hard-easy path.

When we're stressed over long periods of time and our cortisol levels are elevated, we experience a persistent urge to do something. Now. Our brains and bodies tell us that stopping will only escalate the immediate danger. We think that if we stop, we'll drop the ball; things will fall apart the moment we stop holding them together.

But ask yourself honestly, are you really holding everything together, or are you running around with the same exercise trampoline that I carried? Have your efforts so far helped them? Or have they just increased your stress and exhaustion?

Think of the way people speak when they are frightened and

adrenaline has taken hold of them. They rattle on and on—one long run-on sentence of phrases and clauses that all loop back on each other. They define the problem and propose solution after solution. They complain and ask why. They try to find blame in the past and make promises about the future. They keep saying anything and everything to avoid being still and quiet in the uncomfortable present moment. Little of it goes anywhere or makes any sense because, in their panic, they have stopped using punctuation periods.

Grammarians have noted that text messaging has started to make people drop the period from more and more uses, but you can't think *or* communicate clearly without hard stops. The hard stop—the silence at the end of a statement—is as essential to honest and open communication as the words themselves.

When strained, we can also begin to lose the periods in our relationship communication. This can escalate into a frantic outpouring of information and feelings from both sides. When neither of you can pause, neither of you can honor the other's experience, and you lose your connection.

Soon, you are just begging each other to *stop*.

Your person's ability to pause, to stop and think, has been stunted by their substance use. The pathways in their brain have been altered not only by the stress that they want relief from but also by the substance itself.

So, the responsibility to pause falls on you. You are the person with the highest level of consciousness. It's a hard choice, but you can take a pause, a hard stop. You can give yourself space to find new ways of being.

In learning to pause, we can also learn how to resist being reactive to our person's behavior, which allows us to be responsive to their pain. Reacting to our person's behavior keeps us focused on the conflict and differences between us; the focus is on fixing things that are going wrong. It robs us of the time to reflect on our own biases and limitations and how they may be limiting our choices.

Without this reflection, it can be difficult to identify cultural and generational differences that may need to be accepted and honored for the relationship to become safe and strong again. Some of these differences may actually have little to do with substance use.

For example, when family members have strong religious beliefs and practices, seeing loved ones explore different kinds of spiritual practices can feel as unsafe and disordered as substance use.

Some family members are baffled by the career or social choices their person has made, like a son of two highly educated professionals who chooses a traditionally blue-collar career or a daughter who takes steps to permanently opt out of having children.

Some families have even expressed that their loved ones' apparently baffling decisions must have been caused by their SUD. They become, consciously or subconsciously, convinced that substance use has *caused* the other behaviors. Even truly surface-level matters of aesthetics—from clothing choices to tattoos or particular hairstyles—can feel all tied up with substance use. These families come to believe that if they can talk their person back from SUD, they will be able to reverse those other decisions as well.

But that isn't logical. Those associations are tied together in your mind and are interpreted through your own biases, expectations, and limitations. If we react to their behaviors without pausing, we cannot sort out how those limitations are influencing our reactions. That can take us out of alignment with our core values and make it hard to find and honor the connection we want to feel with our person. We become hijacked by our emotional dysregulation that we blame on their behavior.

Silence can be a form of response in itself, and sometimes, it's the best response to a particular behavior. In music, the silence before the musicians play and after the final notes reverberate back into stillness gives the audience the opportunity to absorb what they have heard and fully feel its emotional impact, to *connect* with the heart of the music—to experience the essence of what the music was hoping to convey.

Silence can serve the same beautiful purpose in communication with our loved ones. When we focus on our connection, silence is sometimes all that is needed.

After we lost our home in the fire, a friend of mine took me out for our usual run. Partway through the route, I had to stop. The feelings of loss and displacement became overwhelming, and I disintegrated into a crying mess on the trail.

She was enormously patient with me, and instead of our usual exercise, we went back to the car. We sat in silence for a long time, simply drinking water and eating snacks. There was nothing she could say that would fix what was broken, and I didn't want her to try. I needed her to sit with me in silence. We said hardly anything to each other, but I felt heard. In her patience and quiet, I felt her responsiveness to my pain.

In the long process of recovery, there will be many times that nothing you can say will make it better. Any solution you can provide in a given moment may only provide a modicum of help. Stepping out of providing solutions can be frustrating when you want to solve what feels like a massive problem. But those moments of pause do make a difference, even when all you can offer is being present with someone in silence.

During the span of my son's active addiction, when he could no longer live with us, we were able to establish daily communication, and we met him often. One day that sticks in my memory is when I took him to a gym so he could use the bathroom facilities to shower.

During this time, things were starting to change between us. When he had lived with us, our lives were filled with noise—we yelled and fought and couldn't hear each other over our own needs. At the gym, I brought him soap and a soft towel and waited for him in the lobby while he took care of himself. When he came out freshly showered, he gave me a hug and said simply, "Thank you, Mom."

I accepted his hug and his thanks, but I didn't say anything. Words couldn't provide more in that moment than the support I was already giving. In the quiet, I could take in his thanks and feel it in my heart. In the quiet, he could accept what help I could offer that day to feel a bit more human and loved. Together, we could share our connection in the quiet. It didn't look perfect, but it was one of many moments that allowed us to honor and recenter our connection in our communication and actions toward and for each other.

A pause is not inaction, and silence is not nothing. It's space to breathe and to be and to connect.

Taking a pause can also help escape the cycle of thoughts that keep us trapped in a victim mindset. The victim mindset tells us that we need to find something in the past to blame. We think that finding fault in a single person will save us; it will give us a place to focus in our search for justice. We often fall into this mindset because we've lost sight of everything but the wrongs that seem to consume our lives. From this perspective, the only thing that matters is righting the wrong, finding something or someone to blame so we do not have to look at ourselves.

This is a natural response to the feeling that our situation doesn't make sense. Identifying a villain and a victim allows us to create a simple map of an incredibly complex situation—it gives us clarity of cause and effect, even when things are much messier than this framework suggests.

But the more we look for that bad actor, the less space we give to the current moment. There are many factors that bring any one of us to where we are in the current moment. We may never be able to untangle them all.

The victim mindset can have us reach for hurtful, dismissive language. "I guess you're trying to punish me," "I guess you're abandoning me again," or "I guess my love isn't enough for you." Even as we try to set our reasonable boundaries, the victim mindset can urge us to keep talking and give voice to these hurtful thoughts that prevent us from being heard at all.

It's reasonable to set a boundary around our financial support. But when we fall into the victim mindset, this often comes out as blame: "I can no longer financially support these decisions because you'll just throw it away. I love and want to support you so much, but every time I give you money, all you do is…" This example is an attempt to set a firm and reasonable boundary. However, because this statement goes on and on, the boundary gets lost in the emotional noise of blame and hurt. Our intention is masked by our victim mindset, and our opportunity to be heard is lost.

Instead, we need to pause. We need to get comfortable with silence. We need to use periods. Hard Stops.

"I can no longer financially support these decisions."

Full. Stop.

It's hard to make a stark statement without backloading the emotional whys and hows, but if we want the statement to be heard, we must learn how to stop talking. Otherwise, we are asking to be right, which means someone needs to be wrong. Our person needs boundaries. Our ability to sit with a pause before we speak is what allows the boundary to be heard, to sink in.

Pausing can also allow us to address what we need to *hear* from an interaction as well as what we need to say. It allows us to express what is in our hearts without meanness.

When navigating a relationship with someone with SUD, there are often unknowns and secrets and things they avoid sharing with us or that we avoid asking them. Some of these things do not need to be voiced. If they do not honor our connection, help us develop empathy, or give clarity on things we need to know in order to make decisions, we might not have a right to ask for those things or demand explanations. However, there will be conversations where we need to know things to move forward. The pause can help us listen from a broader perspective to identify those things and understand the differences.

When approaching a difficult conversation with our person, emotional history, resentment, need, hurt, and love can cloud our communication. For instance, consider a conversation where you need to know how money was spent and whether it's gone. Or where a car has been left. Or whether medication has been taken, sold, or is still available somewhere. When we broach these conversations, we are imagining all the possibilities and making assumptions about our person's behavior and reasoning. We've already imagined a dozen answers, among them the worst possible scenarios. When we are in a victim mindset, our minds tell us that our person has already let us down again.

If we do not take a pause, it can be hard to sort out what we need to know from the dark assumptions we are afraid to have confirmed. We may avoid that conversation because we don't want to experience their defensive or aggressive reactions, but this builds resentment and makes the neutral conversation even harder. Taking a pause can allow us to find an emotionally regulated place where we can gather the information we need while keeping our judgment, fears, and resentment at bay.

The victim mindset is an easy-hard path because it exerts energy on everything except taking ownership for how you have participated in coming to this moment and what you can do to move into a better tomorrow. It's easier to fixate on how we have been injured than it is to be present in the current moment and seek understanding. It is even easier to blame our past selves. While it's important to acknowledge patterns and trauma that have affected us in the past, we cannot let it continue to hold us captive there.

In the pause, we can be present in the moment; we can take the hard-easy path. We can create a hard *stop*.

PART THREE

COMMUNICATION

CHAPTER 8

THE ROLE OF REGULATION

EMOTIONAL AND PSYCHOLOGICAL dysregulation is a state of being where a person has difficulty coping with big emotions and patterns of thought. People in a dysregulated state have trouble communicating with others, making clear decisions, remaining calm, and controlling their reactions to negative emotions. Dysregulation encompasses a wide range of disruptive behaviors, including but far from limited to substance use.

Dysregulation stands in the way of connection with others in our lives and can be one of the primary obstacles to recovery. When we attempt to communicate in a state of dysregulation, we are more often speaking through the shadow sides of our values, through our fear and need for control.

When we communicate with our person, dysregulation can color both sides of the conversation. When we understand and account for it, we can make better decisions regarding our communication—not only the words we say but also our physical energy, the boundaries we set, the contexts for conversation, and the things that limit how we can help.

Dysregulation is a term often used in discussing mental health disorders, including SUD, but it is also a state that everyone experiences regularly in their lives. It's not always obvious from a distance. Behaviors like yelling, slamming things, and other disordered behaviors are easy to see as unhealthy. Behaviors like avoidance and deceitfulness can also be dysregulated behaviors that are much harder to see clearly for what they are. Some dysregulated behaviors are invisible, like disordered thinking, negative self-talk, and inner criticism and blame. Professional mental health circles still don't fully understand dysregulation—what causes it, why it affects some more than others, and the range of its expressions—so researchers are still actively studying this emotional state.

However, it is clear that dysregulation can have a wide range of causes, including trauma, stress, and inherited and learned patterns. It does not occur in a vacuum, and in families with SUD, it is likely that many members of the family experience spikes of dysregulation, either chronically or intermittently under stress.

When I try to help families visualize the state of dysregulation, I often sketch a simple diagram. I have grown to think of it as the "Mike Wazowski" diagram because it bears some resemblance to the *Monsters, Inc.* character with his big round head, skinny stick legs, and a shadow circle around the feet.

The circle at the top represents the whole of your healthy being, your truest self. That self includes all of your positive experiences and the positive emotions that go along with them, as well as the negative emotions that follow naturally from life's more difficult experiences. For the self to be unified and whole, it must encompass all of our experiences—good and bad.

When we attempt to compartmentalize so that we do not have to feel and process our negative emotions, sometimes they come out in really big and overwhelming ways. Over time, we can learn how to feel those big emotions and regulate our outward responses to them. We can feel and understand and incorporate them into the whole of our human life and lived experience. It can take time and practice to feel those emotions the way they come to us, not how others want us to feel them, but that agency is essential to the process of learning regulation.

This can be difficult when the feedback and input we receive from others is that those feelings are not valid, should be made smaller or quieter, or are simply incorrect in some fundamental way. When someone denies or diminishes what we are experiencing and the emotions that have arisen in us as a result, we don't feel safe processing and incorporating those feelings into our full selves.

For our feelings to be processed and become part of our cohesive self, they need to be experienced as real in a safe environment, regardless of whether the listener believes them to be real in their mind. When we are not given the opportunity and space to do that, we push the feelings away from us through maladaptive coping skills. To avoid those feelings, we may isolate ourselves, lash out in anger, or use substances to numb the feeling and make it smaller and more acceptable to other people.

These maladaptive coping skills are like fragile lines between us and the big feelings we are pushing away, like the twig-like legs of Mike Wazowski. But these feelings don't really go away; they just never get processed and integrated into our whole human experience in a healthy and cohesive way. We become tethered to them, stuck in them as if we are mired in a puddle of mud.

In this state of dysregulation, all of our actions and the words we choose are stuck in the mud of our unprocessed negative emotions. We are not choosing what represents what *we* really want to say and do with our whole, cohesive selves but only what our fear, anger, and resentment want.

Those emotions don't make good choices. Those emotional choices don't support your connection with your loved ones, honor the balance of your well-being with others, or make real, positive steps toward recovery.

Substance use is a common symptom of dysregulation, and over time, substances can exacerbate the unresolved issues. But substance use is generally not the root *cause* of dysregulation.

This is important to remember because to communicate with empathy, we need to understand that the dysregulation came first. The unprocessed emotions that first caused the dysregulation and triggered the maladaptive coping mechanisms are still there. They are the mud pit the dysregulated person is stuck in.

We may never be able to fully learn or untangle the exact obstacles that caused emotional dysregulation in our loved ones or even in ourselves, but we can learn how to feel and process our emotions in healthier ways that allow us to regulate our nervous system.

When we remain regulated, our whole selves are driving the car, so to speak. Our emotions are felt, but they do not unilaterally determine what we do. Regulation is what allows us to speak calmly when we're angry, stand firm when we're scared, and make clear-headed decisions in difficult circumstances. Regulation also helps show us when we need to step back and create boundaries or distance between ourselves and certain situations or topics of discussion.

There is no one-size-fits-all script for communicating and building the connection between you and your person. When we engage in the process of Parallel Recovery, reflecting on our behavior and keeping what we learned about the brain—and the psychology behind our behavior—in mind, we build a framework that can be a practical and actionable guide for establishing healthy communication with our person. The specific examples of communication in these chapters are intended to demonstrate how that framework works in practice, not as a language model for each individual circumstance but as a general guide for implementing effective communication with your person.

Everybody needs space to speak about what they feel, even people who are using drugs or alcohol. We may not agree with how those feelings are being expressed to us, but we can affirm that we hear them and that the feelings are real.

People who aren't affirmed struggle to know if anything they think or feel is valid. Their dysregulation only deepens through the negative feelings of self-doubt and painful internal criticism. Their inner critic tells them that they don't even know what's right or wrong. That they don't even know how to love somebody. Their internal dialogue makes them feel like they're always wrong, no matter what.

To put it bluntly, I would use drugs, too, if I thought I couldn't do anything right. If I always thought I was letting my friends and family down, I would want to escape that. Anyone would! When we think of it this way, it's easy to understand how substance use becomes such a common problem in our culture. Remembering the dysregulation at the root of substance use and other disordered behaviors allows us to give our loved ones and ourselves more desperately needed empathy and understanding.

When you allow that space and listen to what they are saying with the intention to *understand* without immediately pushing back—needing to be right—you give your person a chance to feel and hear what they are saying themselves and recontextualize it in a safe environment. You are being their support as they take steps toward regulation and, consequently, recovery.

Working toward regulation is something we do for ourselves too. It is not something we can accomplish all at once, and we may experience setbacks. Even in our setbacks, we can ensure we are regulated whenever we communicate with our person in order to make sure we are not making things worse for both of us.

In our contemporary culture, with all its daily technology, there are more and more creative ways to investigate a person's movements and activities than ever before. Tracking location services, AirTags, real-time banking and credit card information, and social media can make gathering information on our loved ones a full-time job.

Most people don't actually want to show up for their loved ones by spying on them. And yet, many families I work with find themselves feeling pushed to do that in their relationships. It's important to understand our drive behind those actions.

We might tell ourselves that we need to know this information, that it is imperative for us to put our energy into gathering that intel and data. If we know these things, we can save them. But more often than not, it is fear driving us to those behaviors and not a need for actionable information.

When you use cell phone location services to find out that your person spent ninety minutes in a strip mall parking lot at 2 a.m., what have you really learned?

You have probably gathered some indirect evidence that supports what you already knew. If you have come to the point of watching that phone dot on your screen, you probably already have a good idea of what is happening. Either they're buying drugs, selling drugs, or doing something that might get them the money to buy drugs. Whatever it is, it's unlikely that anything good is happening in that strip mall parking lot.

Does this mean you'll be able to go to that parking lot and stop what's happening? If your person is an adult, probably not.

Are you going to send a text, all caps and punctuated with profanity, to underscore your feelings on what they are probably doing at that strip mall? You probably already know that a message like that is not going to be received in a way or in a time that will help them. It will only further strain your relationship and reinforce negative patterns.

So what good is knowing that they're in a strip mall parking lot in the middle of the night? Why are you seeking out information that only confirms what you already know?

Your person is out there on their tightrope, and checking your phone repeatedly in the middle of the night is the equivalent of running around with an exercise trampoline. What you're doing is not helping your person, and it is hurting *you*, costing you sleep and peace and keeping you from being able to show up with pause, intention, and connection in mind the next time you see them.

If searching for this information can't lead to making an effective change, what's driving your behavior? The only way to know for certain is to give yourself space to feel what is behind your actions. Often, in the scenarios I encounter in the families I work with, it comes back to fear. Knowing that their person is in that parking lot—or any number of other revealing locations—generates assumptions and fearful possibilities in our minds.

I'm afraid that they will go to jail. That they will get robbed or stabbed or shot. That they will overdose. That they will get sick. That they won't have a future.

Your fear is valid, perhaps even rational, given that those are all possible consequences of their behavior. But I'm sorry to tell you that your fear is also a "you problem."

If you're feeling angry, disappointed, or betrayed, those feelings are valid, just like your person's feelings are valid. But your feelings also belong to you, are a part of you, and are your burden to carry. Spying and angry texts will not prevent your fears from coming to pass. Those behaviors only add to your agitation, feed your anger and resentment, and add fresh layers to your imagined worst-case scenarios. In other words, these coping skills—which serve no constructive purpose—only deepen your dysregulation. When we communicate through that dysregulation, we put our negative emotions on others and add to their burdens and negative experiences. We create a scenario where they are responsible for making us okay.

We have to take hold of those feelings, accept them, and let them become part of our whole human experience before we act. By doing so, we can act with our whole integrated selves and not through the misguided coping mechanisms our fear suggests to us.

When we are regulated, we can also use our understanding to reinforce what we want to see happen for our families and to provide positive affirmation. For example, if your person comes to you and says, "I don't know how to get out of this," you have a lot of choices in how you respond.

A state of dysregulation might tell us to say something like, "You just have to stop" or "Why haven't you…" These reactions are tinged with judgment and criticism. In our impatience for our person to be better, we give instructions that feel out of bounds and unrealistic. Telling someone, "You need to get a job," when their current struggle is getting out of bed only shows that you're really not listening. This makes perfect sense—nobody can really listen from a state of extreme dysregulation.

When we bring ourselves to a calm, grounded place, we can see much more clearly. If our person can't get out of bed, it doesn't make sense to tell them to find a job. A more reasonable response might be to suggest they start by taking a shower. Maybe a slow walk around the block, or maybe we show up with tomato soup and grilled cheese to watch a movie with them and offer no solution, a healthy choice that's actually in reach. With our words, we can acknowledge the weight of what they're feeling and reaffirm the parts of what they are communicating that we want to reinforce and see more of.

"I hear you, and that must be so hard," we might say. "I think, though, what you're saying to me right now is that you understand this is something to get out of. That you want to but haven't found how to. Would you be open to talking to a professional?"

It can be as basic as that in terms of shifting the language we use when addressing SUD and recovery with our loved ones. All of a sudden, you're not taking away their agency or diminishing their feelings. Language that supports their feelings supports their move back toward regulation, where they can make choices with their whole selves and overcome the powerful but destructive patterns of behavior. Language that supports our person's agency is not only kinder, more empathetic, and better for our well-being and connections, but it's simply more effective. No one ever entered recovery and overcame dysregulation because the right person *told them to*. Recovery takes both wanting to recover and having the courage to feel and process those negative emotions in healthier ways.

Supporting that recovery means empowering them to take those steps. In many ways, it doesn't matter exactly what you say but how you say it. Each circumstance is different, and the problems caused by SUD will be specific to the individual.

Empowerment comes through two elements in our communication: the belief and the invitation. We want to show that we believe they can do this. Now, just saying, "You can do this," may not be the way to express that in a believable way.

Imagine you were encouraging someone to climb a ladder. The person is afraid but capable. How would you demonstrate your belief in their ability to climb the ladder? You wouldn't criticize the fact that they haven't just done it already. You wouldn't say, "Why are you afraid? It's just a ladder!" You wouldn't diminish their concerns. These kinds of words and tones communicate the opposite of belief. They suggest astonishment and suggest that you don't really believe they're capable—after all, if you find the task so objectively simple, it's easy for them to feel silly or wrong or broken for finding it so difficult.

What if, instead, you offered to hold the ladder still?

When we truly believe someone can do something, we invite them into the problem-solving process. When communicating with your person about seeking recovery, it is important to give them options and engage their agency in the process so that their steps toward recovery are genuinely their own. Focusing on the invitation shows our belief in them is genuine and allows them to feel and gain support from us.

The specifics of the invitation will depend on the circumstances, but we can't truly know those circumstances unless we listen to their responses and try to meet them where they are. This often means avoiding *why* questions, which are usually triggering and judgmental. "Why haven't you talked to someone?" or "Why did you go back to the parking lot?" Why questions only serve our desire to know and imply an assumption that they have done something wrong: They are wrong, and you are right. This just asks for fights and pushback, and the why just isn't that important.

Instead, we can ask, "What options do you feel like you have? Who have you talked to? Where have you tried to go?"

Asking genuine questions is part of the invitation to start solving the problem. It shows that we really do believe they can do the work of recovery and that we want to support them through supporting *their* choices toward health and recovery, whatever choice is available to them in that direction at that moment.

To overcome a state of dysregulation, we need to safely feel and understand the hard feelings we've repeatedly pushed down. This isn't easy. That's why so many of our easy-hard choices prolong a dysregulated state. Working toward regulation is an ever-continuing journey because we will always have negative experiences and emotions to process. They are part of being alive and active in the world. The more we try to avoid them, to hold them away from our whole and true selves with coping mechanisms that don't work, the more we stay in a dysregulated state. From this state, our actions don't reflect what we really want and value. They don't allow us to show up as the person we want to be for others.

The hard-easy choice toward regulation is the same for both us and our person. When we recognize, name, feel, and accept our emotions as part of us—as our responsibility—we can invite them to do the same and demonstrate our honest belief that we can all recover together.

CHAPTER 9

10,000-FOOT LISTENING

IMAGINE YOU ARE A FARMER. The farm you are cultivating is your whole life. You want it to be fruitful, organized, beautiful, clean, and peaceful. Understandably, you want this farm to grow into its greatest potential.

But sometimes, it's not. Some crops will be harvested sickly, dying, or partly eaten by an insect or an animal. In an attempt to solve the problem, you could spend every moment of your time darting between the rows of plants trying to catch whatever culprit might be causing damage to your crops. You could even fly low over the fields in a crop duster, looking for mice in the field. You may see a mouse or two and be able to catch and prevent a single plant from being eaten, but you wouldn't be able to see the larger infestation—what's really happening.

To understand the problem, you need to take the plane a bit higher to get that 10,000-foot view. Where is the infestation coming from? You need to take a much broader perspective in order to understand the problem, all the areas that it's really affecting, and its true roots.

When working with families to reframe their communication, I turn frequently to the 10,000-foot view, which starts with 10,000-foot listening. Everything has a greater context, including substance use. This approach allows us to understand what's really going on.

When you view the situation from 10,000 feet, you can listen with your whole self and respond to the whole situation. If we lose sight of the bigger picture, we only hear and react to the details. Details aren't important. It's the *circumstances* that matter.

However we communicate, whether through words or actions, we can either be reactive or responsive. When we react, we become hyper-focused on the details. We react because we aren't listening at the 10,000-foot view; we've failed to take in everything with its context. Reactions are knee-jerk, stemming from our instant emotional trigger at the behaviors or words of others. Responses require making full use of the pause. They require us to hold back on immediately giving voice and motion to our reactive thoughts.

For communication to be heard, emotional safety must exist within the relationship. Sometimes, emotional safety requires us to stop talking about how we feel about the details so we can hear the bigger picture, the emotion and context behind the words or actions.

This deliberate stepping back can be so difficult because we're emotionally tied to the problem. We're scared. In the case of family, we feel compelled to react because our family members' pain feels like our own. But it is not our pain; it is theirs.

There are three basic tools we can use to ensure we are communicating in a way that can be genuinely heard, even in difficult circumstances and relationships. When considering these three tools, remember that this is not a script. I cannot give you the words to say, only the strategies for choosing your own.

In case you're tempted to look for a script, let me offer a word of caution. Coming into a conversation with a script is a surefire way to signal that you are not there to listen but to *manage*. Reciting phrases or questions in careful ways that do not acknowledge the context is not a way to step into your relationship or honor your connection with your person. The examples throughout this chapter are amalgams of instances I and the families I have worked with have experienced, along with hypothetical extensions. They are all intended to show how these listening and communication strategies can work in practice rather than suggesting specific words to use.

The first tool is to listen with empathy. This is where we take our 10,000-foot view. Remembering that our person is a full and separate whole, we take our step back and try to understand. When we want to understand something, we ask authentically curious questions. We ask what and how, open-ended questions that seek out data and understanding without imposing limits on the answers we want. We ensure that we can really listen to our person's responses, not the responses that *we* want to hear.

We also exhibit open listening by being present with our body language and posture. If we're not in a position to do this, it is better to ask to communicate at a different time. When we pretend to be present, "uh-huh-ing" and nodding our way through a conversation that needs our engagement, we only harm the relationship by reinforcing that we are not emotionally safe or available.

Genuinely curious questions are open-ended and not packed with expectations, commentary, judgment, or limits to the conversation. Genuinely curious questions invite genuinely honest answers—even when that honesty is hard to hear. "How can you use drugs when you know how bad they are for you?" is a loaded question, not a curious one. Curious questions ask, "When you are having a hard time, what is going through your mind?"

If you do have suggestions or thoughts you want to note, ask permission to share them: "Hey, so you've just given a lot of information, and I have some thoughts." Then you might say, "Would you be open to hearing them?"

Be prepared to hear—and respect—a "no." The only response then is to say, "Okay, when and if you'd like to hear about them, let me know, and I'll be happy to share." This creates emotional safety in your relationship by showing you can listen and that they have agency in how they give and receive information.

The second tool is to reflect and validate what they communicate with you. If we try to minimize or lessen what is being expressed to us, we demonstrate that we are not safe to communicate with, which damages our connection and, ultimately, our ability to create influence. That does not mean we have to agree with everything our person says, condone their behavior, or support their choices. In reflecting their communication back to them, we show that we hear and understand them and that we believe their emotions are real and difficult to feel.

The third tool is empowerment. We communicate "I believe you can do this" with words and actions that support that genuine belief and invite our person to take the lead in their own problem-solving. This requires us to step out of the mindset of "but they aren't doing this!" and step into the belief that they actually can do this.

Keeping these tools in mind can guide us in choosing words that honor our connection to them and their autonomy while reinforcing positive steps to recovery.

Communication is like playing catch. It involves a back-and-forth pattern. You have to be engaged in listening to catch what they are saying, and to be willing to engage with the conversation at their level. You need to be able to toss the ball back in a way that allows your person to catch it.

This seems easy enough, but it can get hard. We often hear things we don't want to accept. When that happens, it's as if your person tossed you a ball you don't want to catch. You don't even want to touch it. It's been chewed up by the dog. It's deflated, dirty, and covered in slobber or some other unidentifiable slime. You may hate that they've chosen to play the game with this ball, or even play this game at all, but the only way to keep connecting with them is to toss it back for them to catch.

You might feel compelled to say, "You know what, I have a nice ball in the garage. Let's play with that instead." But they started a game with you. This is the game—slimy ball and all—that they are able to play right now. If you try to control the game by enforcing your ball standards, you communicate that you're not willing to engage with them except on your terms.

That doesn't mean you have to enjoy catching that slimy ball. And, in fact, that ball may be very difficult to catch. A dysregulated person may feel that everything bad in their lives is the responsibility of someone else, and that is what they express. The ball they toss to you is that their boss, teacher, partner, peers, doctor, psychologist, or neighbor hates them, is against them, and is making everything unfair for them. That's the ball they are choosing to play with in this moment. Validating that feeling by engaging in the game doesn't mean you agree with their assessment objectively; it only means you're validating the way things feel to them right then. If they do not feel heard for what they are experiencing, they cannot step out of that belief and see another perspective.

In this case, tossing the ball back might sound like, "That sounds overwhelming. I'm not sure how I would handle that. What are you thinking?"

In this way, we're not reacting to how *we* feel about what they're saying and feeling. We're listening and looking for the bigger picture and trying to understand. It will probably suck, but this is the ball they chose, and we can't choose differently for them. If we try to substitute the ball, we invalidate how they feel about the situation, which makes the game of the conversation emotionally unsafe for them. We also can't gloss over what they say with platitudes and dismissals. We can't diminish what they say with our words any more than we can put what they're feeling in our pocket and take it away with us, saving them from the reality of their experience. Painting that gnarly ball pink and putting a smiley face sticker on it isn't any better than trying to substitute a new ball.

Other times, we might struggle to catch the ball because our person asks for a "solution"—the thing that is "all that they need" to fix everything in their lives.

All I need is a car, a job, to pay off this debt, to move into a new apartment...

When someone we love tosses that ball to us, it's very hard to catch. It's even harder to toss it back unchanged. It is very tempting to many of us to then toss that solution back by giving them what they asked for. We probably have fifty solutions for these "all I need" problems because they are usually small, solvable issues.

Use my car this week. Uncle Rob says you can work in his store. Here's some money to pay down your credit card. There's a place on Nice Street; I'll pay the first three months' rent...

Here we are again with our useless exercise trampoline, trying to catch them.

This reaction is an easy-hard path because those "solutions" don't address the underlying problems, only the symptoms. Our person may show up prepared to do solution gymnastics—*all I need is X, Y, and Z*—but this only pushes the real opportunity for change down the road. We feel like we can provide something easily that will help, so we do and hope that it really will make the hard problem go away. But the real, hard truth of their reality can't be realized through a series of band-aids and short-term fixes. The hard reality of their situation is that they are the ones who must address the underlying problem responsible for the solutions that are no longer working. They need to step forward into real solutions. Recognizing the reality of that is an opportunity for real, lasting change. Tossing back a quick fix to the immediate small problem only delays that reckoning.

The hard-easy path in these scenarios is not to toss everything they asked for but to toss that old ball back to them as it is. Validate that what they're dealing with is a hard thing and ask them what solution they think they need. Ask them what their options are, who they have spoken to, and what they have tried.

Eventually, they may look down at the ball you've given back to them and see it for what it is. This gives them the opportunity to recognize their reality and step toward their own solution—where and how they are going to get a different ball. You may then choose to step forward as well, be engaged with their solution, and offer to support them how you can. But you are not the architect of that solution—they are.

This honors their autonomy and responsibility for their problems, and it also keeps you out of the potential "bad guy" role down the line. It isn't likely that giving your person what they asked for will solve the problem. And if you propose a different solution that then doesn't solve the problem—or worse, turns into a new problem —you become another person to blame. The next time they toss you a ball, it may be even more unappealing than the slimy one, something like: "I did what you told me to do and look where it got me."

But if your person is the architect of that solution, gradually, they will realize that the next solution is their responsibility too. When everyone else avoids the position of "bad guy," your person will no longer be able to point fingers and be faced with a mirror instead. They will be left to examine themselves and their role in the problem. They will be left to consider why their options are limited. They will be left to experience the truth of their condition and see what paths are open for them to take, however hard they might be.

This is not a crisis-level strategy for communication; this is a *forever* strategy for communication. Whether your person is in active addiction, contemplating recovery but not yet committed, in treatment, or in recovery and sober, supporting the relationship with thoughtful, responsive communication will always be the best way to maintain a positive and loving connection. Listening with the 10,000-foot view always allows for that communication to be healthy and rooted in positive connection.

One family I worked with struggled with the decisions their son was making in recovery. Though he was soberly choosing things in his life, to his family, the choices felt like consequences of his struggle with SUD that he shouldn't have to pay now that he was in recovery. The family, for several generations, were all educated, white-collar professionals. For their son, college had been a difficult time, and during a time of active substance use, he had dropped out. In recovery, he chose not to go back but to pursue a trade apprenticeship program instead. In communicating this with his family, they had a hard time accepting this as a positive solution. It simply wasn't the vision they had for their son, and they reacted to the news with how they felt about the choice rather than being responsive to the greater context of what their son was communicating to them.

In a session following this conversation with their son, I asked them if they'd asked him why he'd made that choice and what he found attractive about the trade program.

They said they had and summarized his responses. He didn't want to sit through lectures anymore; he didn't want to risk having access to loan money; he didn't want to spend the years it would take; he didn't want...he didn't want...he didn't want....

The way they summarized the son's response was very telling, because those are *not* answers to the question "Oh, what sounds good about that? Tell me more about it." Those are answers to the question "Why aren't you going back to college?" That question focuses on the negative and limits his potential answers to the framework *they* wanted to set for his life. It doesn't show genuine curiosity but imposes the desire to bring back that future image they had for him when he was a teenager, a ship that had long since sailed.

"Why aren't you..." can become a habit of communication that becomes ingrained so deeply we can't even see it. We might intend to be curious and ask why, but it comes out "Why aren't you..." when we are not actively listening with our 10,000-foot view.

During active substance use, we might be tossed some unattractive balls to play catch with, and the question "Why aren't you using a better ball?" seems like the only logical response. But "Why aren't you . . ." is diminishing and dismissive, no matter where your person is or what kind of ball they're tossing you.

In the case of this family, this type of question became such a habit that they couldn't see the positive in what their son was communicating to them. It wasn't a nasty deflated baseball, but a different kind of ball altogether—a football, a whiffle ball, an unripe cantaloupe—and they still reacted to how they felt about the change rather than trying to understand what was and would be appealing about the change for their son.

Remaining responsive rather than reactive keeps us from making things worse. There may be times when the ball that we don't want to catch is our person telling us about a mistake they made. It might be a big or a small mistake, and they might own it as their mistake, or they may put it off onto something or someone else or just distance themselves from the mistake. The most common sentence in passive voice, after all, is "mistakes were made."

Because we love them, our person's mistake may hurt us and provoke negative reactions and thoughts. They lost a gift we gave them, or they failed to manage their time properly and won't be able to keep their commitments, or they did something that embarrasses us. It may be a bigger mistake—they lost their job or were injured in carelessness or recklessness. Or perhaps they relapsed.

If, when catching that ball, we react to it, we might blurt out something about how ugly the ball is, how hard it is to catch, or how they never would have tossed you that ball in the first place if they weren't so disorganized, thoughtless, or otherwise broken.

That reaction only causes harm. Now, in addition to dealing with the mistake, they will be carrying the hurt we've passed back to them. There is a time, place, and way to express our feelings, but it is not reactionary nor in the moment.

Instead, we can choose to ask, "What will you do about that now?" and toss the ball back to them.

That invites them to tell us how they will replace what they lost or deal with the small or big problem caused by the mistake. In the case of return to use, it invites them to recommit and share how they need support.

No matter the context, there is always a possibility that we will be tossed a ball we desperately do not want to catch. We may want to react to this slimy ball hurtling toward us, but reaction is not engagement, and it is certainly not connection. To be responsive in the relationship, we pause to feel and process our emotions, we listen to what is behind our person's words, and we meet them where they are instead of where we wish they were.

CHAPTER 10

BOUNDARIES VS. RULES

DISAGREEMENTS CAN BE common in any family, but in families affected by SUD, they can be intense and frequent. Navigating arguments is often the first skill families want to learn. In the process of navigating conflict-ridden relationships, forming clear, consistent, and predictable boundaries is an essential tool. But boundaries can be tricky when we are in the midst of a disagreement. In heated situations, the focus should be on de-escalating conflict in the moment and protecting your wellness. Too often, this gets confused with the idea of "winning" the fight.

Instead, think of boundaries as a tool to draw lines around the topics and habits that create tension. When you create boundaries for the purpose of letting others understand how they can be in your emotional or physical spaces, you can stay in the conversations that are essential to maintaining a connection with your person while avoiding conflicts.

For instance, imagine a relationship between a brother and sister. Whenever a disagreement begins, the brother turns to name-calling. He often calls his sister a coward or references her fear in another way that suggests inherent weakness. This is a sensitive point for her, and in her natural but misguided attempts to prove herself, she frequently escalates disagreements into arguments.

To break this cycle, the sister may—in a moment of relative calm—reflect for herself on why she participated in escalating the conflict. Recognizing that this is a sensitive point for her, she communicates this with her brother. She may think that this is setting a boundary, but it is missing crucial elements. She has made a good first step in reflecting on her behavior, especially if she does so with the genuine intent of avoiding future conflict and connecting with her brother where he is. But in attempting to set a boundary, what she has actually done is set a rule, which is doomed to backfire.

The next time the brother tells her that she's "nothing but a scared little girl," she yells back, "I have told you that you can't say things like that to me!" Rather than a tool to de-escalate, the rule has become a way to win the fight. She reflected on her needs and the context of her reactions, but she did not follow through with healthier responses. The two are still trapped in the reactionary cycle of the conflict.

In this case, the sister wants to use the boundary she *tried* to draw as a rule to control his behavior and thinking. What she really wants is to keep him from *thinking* that way about her. She wants him to validate her self-image. She tries to enforce this rule to make that happen. Unfortunately, rules rarely control or change another person's beliefs or actions. All we can control is our reactions.

What is a more effective way of protecting herself from the word attacks from her brother? Rather than hurling the "rule" at her brother like a weapon, she simply needs to hold the line as a genuine boundary. This requires both another layer of communication and a genuine willingness to calmly follow through. When expressing to her brother how this affects her, she can add that she will not participate in discussions where it escalates to such name-calling and that she will end the conversation if it does.

In this case, when her brother resorts again to calling her

cowardly or weak, she doesn't escalate the conversation into conflict but follows through with her spoken intention to step away.

"I have said that I cannot continue conversations when you call me names like that," she might say. "We are clearly not ready to have this conversation, so let's try again another day." She can then remove herself physically from the conversation—rising from the table or hanging up the phone—communicating that she means what she says.

This is not an easy thing to do. The easy-hard path is forming the rule—telling him to stop and hoping he will respect her wishes so that she won't have to change the way she responds. The hard-easy path, the only way forward into true connection, is defining what her response will be and following through when the occasion arises.

The term "boundaries" has crossed over from therapy sessions to mainstream popular use, and like most terms do when they trend on Google and social media, it has lost much of its meaning and nuance. There's no real way to control the changing meaning of popular terms in the broader social landscape, and if some choose to invoke the term to block people on social media or sell self-care planners, more power to them. But because of its growing and frequently more casual use, for our purposes, it may help to clearly define what setting healthy boundaries looks like by first outlining what it isn't.

Boundaries are not bargaining chips or tricks to win arguments. They are not impermeable walls you set around yourself to insulate you from any potential hurt or responsibility.

Setting boundaries is frequently conflated with the "detach with love" style of counsel, but setting boundaries is not about detachment. In detachment, there is no need for boundaries because you have stepped out and away.

In fact, boundaries are not about creating distance at all. Setting boundaries is about finding ways to stay connected safely without sacrificing your needs and autonomy. Boundaries allow us to step into relationships, not out.

Communicated properly, boundaries are also not a strategy to change others' behavior. They can be tools to help guide communication when relationships get difficult, but they do not work as ultimatums or leverage to force your person to change. When they are formed with that intention, they not only lead to resentment on both sides, but they also won't work.

Boundaries are not about controlling contexts outside yourself. They are about communicating clear expectations for your actions in response to situations. No matter how much you love your person, you cannot control their behavior. But that doesn't mean you have to accept any treatment they give you, take up responsibilities that should not be yours to bear, or sacrifice your space, safety, or any dimension of your well-being.

When you communicate clear boundaries, you invite your person to connect with you in a way where you both can offer and receive love. Instead of "You can't, unless..." boundaries are about "*We can*, if..."

This distinction may be difficult to feel in the specific contexts of your relationships, but holding it clear in your heart and mind as you choose boundaries for yourself will ensure that they are made with honest intentions, which in turn makes them much easier to hold and keep up with through the long term.

⁂

Before you can set boundaries, you need to understand *why* you're setting those boundaries. As I've said before, there's no script for genuine relationships. Each individual is unique, so each relationship between individuals is doubly so. In turn, it is up to you to design your boundaries based on your life, your needs, and your relationships. I cannot outline for you a set of one-size-fits-all boundaries. They are contingent on your values, your circumstances, and the singular connection you share with your person.

Your connection with your person is what is of most importance. Their behavior makes up the details—the circumstances—of the connection. The behaviors associated with SUD can be scary and damaging; SUD can lead people we love to lie, steal, manipulate, and damage their environments out of an extension of their self-harm. Since those behaviors can hurt you and the connection you share, you may need to create physical or emotional distance from those behaviors. But that is *not* the same as creating distance from your *person*.

To create distance from the behavior, remember that the relationship is based on what's important to you about this person. Ask yourself, *Who are they?* And not, *What are they doing?*

Boundaries are lines around what you will accept while you are communicating with your person or when that person is in your home. If you share a home with them, the lines can blur easier around boundaries that can feel like rules about what a person can or cannot do in their own spaces or to their bodies.

There are few situations where you can implement *rules* in a relationship with someone. When the person is an adolescent under your care, rules are appropriate. There may be rules when there is an imminent threat of danger or causing harm to others, like when substances are in reach of young children or when people drive while intoxicated. When rules are broken, there can be consequences, but it's important to understand that these consequences may not be effective at changing behavior. The justice system is full of people who violate rules—laws—willingly and knowingly. Many of us violate rules when we don't see the value in them. Rules can be used when necessary, but they are not a path toward connection in a relationship.

Boundaries set expectations about *your* behavior in particular situations. Rules try to set expectations about *others'* behavior.

Since you can't control others' behavior, creating rules is often a fool's errand.

But drawing the boundary isn't the hard part. The hard part is following through with it. Just because you draw the boundary doesn't mean it will be respected. And if it is not, you should follow through with your planned response. Following through requires being prepared to actually follow through.

Some boundaries may be harder to draw than others because some of our wellness needs are less concrete and obvious than others. If we consider the eight dimensions of wellness (emotional, physical, occupational, social, spiritual, intellectual, environmental, and financial), some of them can be more clearly observed and measured than others. Your physical and environmental wellness, for instance, can be adversely affected by second-hand smoke, so that is a clear place to draw a boundary. Your occupational wellness can be defined by the existing boundaries of your workplace and career needs.

To maintain a boundary here, you might establish clear expectations about your time. For instance, if it is disruptive for you to answer calls or texts during working hours, you can clearly communicate that you will not answer during work hours and will return calls when you get home. And then you stick to it—don't answer your phone during those hours. For your own sake, don't even let it ring if that sparks feelings of guilt or obligation. Hearing it might perpetuate the narrative that they must need you right now, but this thinking keeps us trapped in a reactionary cycle.

I understand that boundaries like this one are difficult for some to keep. It is tempting to add caveats like "only call me at work during an emergency," but dysregulated people—including many of those affected by SUD—may have a distorted view of what constitutes an emergency. Others just exist in a constant state of near-emergency. But issues caused by their use and their choices and behavior are their responsibility to respond to. You can still be available in the times that work for your life and wellness for help and support, but putting your job in jeopardy to meet their constant needs is going to cause greater harm down the road for everyone. In actual emergencies, you should not be the one to call anyway. There are professionals for that.

Your financial security may boil down to literal math. Put limits on what you're able to provide and stick to them. If this boundary feels hard to keep, revisit your core values and consider whether the shadow sides of those values are showing up in that struggle. Your need to be needed, or the belief that being a provider means an *endless* provider, can also keep you trapped in that reactionary loop.

Your emotional, spiritual, and intellectual wellness, being internal and personal to you, are harder to protect because it's harder to define your needs for those areas. But these areas are no less important to your well-being. To define your emotional, spiritual, and intellectual needs, you may need to revisit the soul searching I outlined in part one. When you can find your core values and understand how the shadow sides of those values may be showing up in your behavior, choices, and communication, you can create boundaries around your inner world with greater intention.

You may be afraid of how your person will react to your boundaries. When holding a boundary requires putting physical distance between you, families often worry that their people will say they feel abandoned. Our fear of their reaction can stem partly from our need for validation. Our need for validation leads us to believe that, as they say, we are "abandoning" them.

When someone is dysregulated, they are not a good source of validation for others, so putting and keeping your need for validation on someone who can't provide it continues a cycle that keeps you both entangled in a desperate web. Stepping out of that cycle is a move toward recovery for you both. Remember that your person can choose to agree with the boundary or not. You are simply following through on what you said you would do in a particular circumstance.

There is still no script, but the words you use to communicate your boundaries matter to their success. What might feel like semantics—just a different way to communicate the same idea—is actually a reflection of a very important difference in your intention and how well you can be heard.

One way this can show up is through phrasing like "I love you, but..." I caution you not to use this particular structure to communicate your boundaries. "But" is a turning word; it negates, qualifies, gives conditions, and lessens everything that comes before it. Nothing after the word "but" matters as much as how significantly that word maims what comes before—in this case, "I love you." Anything heard after the but puts conditions on love.

"I love you, and..." provides a way to stay connected while protecting your wellness. What follows is an invitation to find a context that works for you both. Regardless of the particular words you choose, remember that *invitation* should be at the heart of your communication, including your communication of boundaries.

Words from people we love tend to penetrate us, and that is where the danger to our emotional, intellectual, and spiritual wellness comes from. We can't control what they say, but we can communicate which topics and modes of conversation we will engage with and which will result in our physical distance.

When there is conflict in conversation that escalates to cursing and anger-driven language, we can feel attacked. In that moment, we may not be able to continue the conversation in a way that would make us feel proud, in control of ourselves, and loving. This is a natural reaction, but we can take advantage of the pause and choose to remove ourselves from the conversation rather than escalate it. Boundaries provide us the opportunity to communicate how we will respond before the escalation ever starts.

When defining boundaries, keep the commentary and direction of your words on yourself, on what you feel, need, and will do.

In this way, you are distinguishing your boundaries from attempts to control. You maintain an open invitation to connect as long as the context remains agreeable to both of you. You are telling them, "This is how I can love you and myself at the same time."

We may also find that particular topics and modes of conversation cause us emotional harm. Our family members may have ideas that we not only disagree with but even hearing about them—especially ad nauseum or in a rant—can be harmful to the relationship. Ideas about religion, politics, different social groups, or belief systems run deep and affect our core values about right and wrong. When we set a boundary around such topics and make it clear that we cannot hold a conversation centered around them, it's important to follow through—leave the table or hang up the phone if the topic comes up and your person refuses to drop it.

We do not have to choose to be whipping posts for beliefs that are abhorrent to us. We communicate boundaries to set expectations. And we follow through to make it clear that we have set our boundaries thoughtfully and with intention. A simple statement of "This is a topic I will not discuss. Is there anything else you want to talk about?" lets them know how you can continue the connection.

Sticking to boundaries takes practice; it's a bit like building a muscle. Whether our instincts have previously led us to be controlling or overly accommodating, redrawing those lines and habits takes time. When you shift a mindset, you begin to understand the necessity and value of boundaries. Give yourself permission to start small. You don't have to redraw territory all at once, but you can find ways to start modeling standards for your safety and wellness.

When you find something you can stick to, that you can commit to keeping as a boundary, then you can make progress in the relationship by showing that commitment, no matter how small the boundary is. It is a way of communicating through repetition and steadfastness that you mean what you say when you say it.

One family I worked with struggled to form and keep boundaries with their young adult son. He lived with them, and his behavior was continuing to escalate and become more and more dangerous, not only for himself but for them by extension. Understandably and importantly, the parents were not ready to require him to leave their home permanently. He was so young, and they worried what would happen if he were on his own. But there are many options besides tolerating harmful behavior and telling someone to find a new place to live. You can put other boundaries in place to take back some of your peace. That's what worked for this family.

We started small. In this household, the mom cooked dinner every night. She enjoyed doing this for her family and saw it as an expression of love. But as many women know, the acts of service we do for our families can become taxing when they are unappreciated or disrespected. Their son's behavior was increasingly erratic, and they never knew exactly when he would be home, nor in what state. As we talked about this part of their problem, I suggested making it known that everyone in the household would need to let her know by three o'clock if they were coming home for dinner. If she didn't hear from a particular family member, she would not make dinner for them.

At first, this mom resisted setting this boundary. She liked to cook, after all, so dinner wasn't a big deal. I reminded her that this was true—dinner *isn't* a big deal—and that went for her and her son. When there was a fridge, a pantry full of food, and a drive-thru on the corner, no one was going to starve. And the request wasn't unfair, unreasonable, or difficult. It was about meaning what she said so that she could stop living with and expressing the resentment that formed daily.

Of course, the family had many issues that were bigger than dinner. And all of them would be helped by her demonstrating that she meant what she said and she could follow through on her boundaries. If "no" always means "maybe," then "no" loses all impact. We need to learn how to draw a line for ourselves and keep it by saying no when someone crosses it. Sometimes, we have to start small in order to build the ability to hold our line.

Very soon after she implemented this boundary, her son came home unexpectedly. He had not told her he would be home for dinner. She had made hamburgers that night, but she hadn't made one for her son. When he came into the dining room, he asked, "Where's mine?"

"Oh gosh," she said. "You didn't tell me by three, so I assumed you wouldn't be here. Feel free to make yourself something, and if you let me know tomorrow by three, I'd be happy to include you."

He was dysregulated, so his reaction was overblown, to say the least. He threw a chair and screamed nasty and hurtful things.

She didn't make him a hamburger.

The next day, he let her know he'd be home for dinner.

Making a hamburger might not seem like a big deal, but saying no and *meaning it* is important to establish a healthy relationship that includes respecting yourself and your needs. You can manage your fear about your person's potential reactions when you are certain that the request is not unreasonable, controlling, or genuinely harmful.

If you resist following through on small boundaries, they have a way of being pushed back. The problems in the relationship and environment can continue to escalate with every "maybe" that means "yes" and every "no" that means "maybe." Eventually, if you have not been setting and keeping your hamburger boundaries in place, we can get to a place where our anger, resentment, and emotional and even physical safety are such a risk that there's no way forward without first creating a significant distance, up to and including asking them to no longer be in your home at all. This may feel like a drastic step, but it is one that can be hopefully avoided if clear boundaries have supported the relationship along the way.

Setting a boundary doesn't always mean that it will be respected. If, for instance, you set a boundary around giving your person money, you cannot assume that they will stop asking. In fact, you should be prepared to assume that they will continue to ask. Remember, boundaries are about *your* behavior, not theirs. Following through on the boundary means saying no as many times as it takes. When you tire and say yes, you reinforce that no actually means maybe. You have to do the work of maintaining the boundary for as long as it serves you; it is not their work but yours.

One of the hardest areas to form boundaries around is your home, especially with adult children. When your home is also their home, it can be difficult for you to be the one that puts physical distance between you and their harmful behavior.

When an adult lives with you in your home, it's their home too. When an adult lives with you, even if that adult is your grown child, you have invited them into an agreement with you. Agreements are collaborative and mutual, not dictated. Behaviors that make you uncomfortable in your shared home must be measured and understood differently than when a person visits you in your home.

When a person who does not live with you uses substances, you can invite them to spend time in your home with conditions. You can say to them, "It is too hard to see you intoxicated. We love you, and we want you with us. What time of day is better for you?" If the person then comes to your home impacted by drugs or alcohol, you can simply say, "It doesn't seem like this is a good time. I am uncomfortable with how you are behaving. Let's catch up tomorrow on the phone."

That kind of invitation can genuinely work because even in the deepest depths of SUD, people do want to be loved more than they want that substance. It may not look picturesque, it may only be for a couple of hours at an inconvenient time, but being able to maintain that conditional invitation keeps the connection alive. That connection can be the motivation that they need to get better, but only if they can step into it and accept the invitation through their own choices.

This is much more difficult in a shared home. When you

attempt to set a "boundary" about what an adult can put in their bodies in their own home—and when you're not willing to follow that boundary through to a logical conclusion—you set your communication up to fail. This just adds to the cycle of resentment, keeping the whole family sick.

Many parents of adult children with SUD are simply not ready to draw a boundary whose conclusion would be to tell their child to find somewhere else to live. No one can tell a parent when it's time for that step.

One of the best ways to avoid that eventuality is to start smaller. Find your hamburger and protect your peace in whatever ways you can. Soul-searching and reflection are central to creating healthy boundaries. That's the reason this chapter comes later in this book and not in the first or second chapter. Boundaries are important—they are, in fact, crucial—but they can't necessarily come first.

CHAPTER 11

COLLABORATIVE AGREEMENTS

THE PATH of recovery is not linear—neither for those directly affected by SUD nor their families.

There was a long period of time for my family where it seemed that every step we took in a healthy direction came with several steps back. Our son was living with us, but none of us were living in peace. There had been several attempts at treatment, some more promising than others, but he was still in active addiction. Our house felt chaotic, with daily screaming matches and holes punched in walls. Sometimes, I tried to grab a little peace by slamming a door shut. But of course, that's not peace at all; it's just a desperate, misguided grab for some sense of control. When I slammed a door, the yelling would cut off, and my brain would reward me for stopping the onslaught. I knew better. Slamming the door was just the easy-hard choice. The chaos was still there, waiting, muted only for a moment.

Eventually, I realized that *I* had to change in order for things to truly get better. We had to set—and *stick to*—boundaries that worked for us, where we could carve out a sense of genuine peace that would give us the choice to move toward each other.

For us, that meant we could no longer live together under one roof.

Over time, we achieved small victories toward healthier connections with each other. And soon, those victories came with real steps forward for all of us. Finally, we had stopped the dance of desperate, unsupported attempts to move forward that were always doomed to fall back.

There came a time when our new way of engaging with each other was tested with a major challenge. Our son had been in long-term treatment, with over eight months of continuous sobriety. He video-called my husband and me, and it was immediately clear that something was happening. From the video call, we could clearly see the distinctive shape of an airplane window behind him.

"Why does it look like you're on a plane?" I asked him.

He took a breath and said, "Because I am. I bought a one-way ticket to Utah. I'm moving."

My husband and I looked at each other, stunned.

Leaving the treatment center—a place where he had been making progress—was not what we would have chosen for him. It brought up scary memories for my husband and me. We had seen so many relapses where we didn't know where he was or what he was doing, and those periods felt terrifyingly uncertain.

But this wasn't like that, and we had to recognize that. He wasn't running away. This wasn't a relapse. He wasn't in some dark place where we could only imagine the choices he was making. He was on a plane. He'd made a choice, and he was sharing it with us.

It was a challenge for us to hear it. And challenges are genuine opportunities to show that your growth is real.

In talking with our son, we listened as he told us about his decision. The treatment center had tried to keep him there and had told him that this decision was tantamount to a relapse. They gave him the message that this choice was giving up on his recovery and said, "Let us know when you're ready for help again," as he was on his way out the door.

But he was ready for something different.

He told us he had already spoken to two sober living places in Utah, and he gave us their contact numbers. He acknowledged that he would need to find a therapist and would probably need help finding one in his new city. He told us this all from a spirit of collaboration—sharing his decisions and concerns.

We had spent so long working together on our relationship and connection, and we had finally moved past the point of us telling him what he could or could not do. At this point, our relationship had evolved from choosing combativeness to collaboration. We had finally reached a point of empowerment and partnership. He was not *asking* for our help but rather inviting us to choose whether we were going to partner with him in these new decisions or not. We had built our boundaries, and he had gotten used to hearing no. He knew there was a chance that we would say no to this request, too, and that he would have to find different ways to get what he needed. He was opening the conversation up to a possible new agreement between us.

Although his choice surprised us, we managed to put aside our need for the safety of the known and validate that moving to Utah was not the same as a relapse. We acknowledged that it wasn't what we would have chosen for him, but because we were partnering with him—not doing *for* him—we wanted to support him as he figured out this new life step. So, we asked him what he thought he would need to be successful.

Because we had done the work to hand over his recovery to him and work on our own recovery process, he was prepared for the question and was ready to define his needs.

Later, we spoke to the therapist at his previous treatment center, and he was certain that nothing positive could come from our son's decision. "Whelp," he told us, "I guess we're back to square one."

We didn't feel back at square one, whatever "square one" really meant. Everything our son told us sounded like he was trying to build a healthy life. He wasn't throwing in the towel on his recovery. While he was picking a less linear route to an outcome than we would have preferred, he was not leaving treatment to go back to active addiction.

This was my first experience in recognizing that professionals—as amazing, knowledgeable, and helpful as they can be—don't always have all the answers.

We told the therapist that his interpretation didn't coincide with the conversation we had just had with our son. "It's not the plan we would have laid out for him," I told him. "But he's twenty years old, and he can make his own decisions. This is *his* plan. What we are hearing from him right now is that he's willing to stay sober and acknowledge what support he'll need. He's asking that we walk alongside him and support him, however we're willing to do so. That's not square one at all. In fact, this doesn't feel like anywhere we've been before."

His now-former therapist didn't have much to say to that.

For this agreement to work, we had to be in a place where we could approach it together. That wouldn't have worked if we hadn't done the work of setting boundaries and understanding our own patterns and needs. Boundaries come before agreements for two reasons.

First, boundaries are about you. They are borders around what you need for your emotional and physical well-being. When our well-being feels under attack and we are trapped in dysregulation, we can't see or think clearly enough to make collaborative agreements with others. Boundaries give us the space to become a person who is emotionally safe to communicate with. That doesn't mean we always agree with what our person says or that they will always agree with what we say; it just means that we're clear and consistent with our communication. Our yeses are yeses, and our nos are nos, both through our words and our actions.

Secondly, agreements are collaborative. Boundaries are set without consultation—they are *your* decisions about *your* actions.

Agreements, on the other hand, come from both parties. There's a fifty-fifty split between considering your needs and considering theirs. Before collaboration can occur, more likely than not, you've done some hamburger work. You've practiced clarity and communication in smaller stakes.

When you have done the work of maintaining your boundaries while still honoring the connection between you, the relationship can shift toward mutual trust. That doesn't necessarily mean you're on the same page about everything; trust just means you're building a connection based on predictability and reliability. In a state of dysregulation, reliability and stability may be out of reach for your person, but you can model the safety of trust in the context of your relationship with them. This can open the path to influence because as your person sees your willingness and ability to change, it opens up the possibility of them changing too.

In the safe spaces created by boundaries, we can find predictability and common ground. Boundaries are not necessarily permanent or forever, but when they're set, they should be considered set in stone. They should only be changed when the circumstances have changed so significantly that the boundary is no longer necessary to protect your emotional or physical well-being. The bar for that change should be set very high. And it's possible that some boundaries may never "come down" because their need continues.

Agreements are different because they are collaborations between two parties. They should be organic and fluid to see what works for both parties over time. They can continuously evolve to fit both of your changing needs and circumstances. Understanding agreements in this light helps avoid resentment and misunderstanding.

When families are supportive and involved in SUD treatment, it becomes staggeringly more effective. Most families are more than willing to support treatment—some are eager and even desperate for it—but the reality of the treatment, especially treatment as it exists and is available in our country, often requires significant financial support.

Financial support, such as providing funds for treatment or offering the use of a vehicle, is a great opportunity for creating agreements. Coming to that support through an agreement invites their participation, which decreases resentment and increases empowerment and accountability.

Financial support that doesn't have clearly communicated parameters in an agreement can lead to resentment and poorly used funds. When support is established as part of an agreement, not only are you providing direct help that works with your needs, but your person also has skin in the game, so to speak. Though you are providing material to make treatment possible, *they* are making active choices and steps in their recovery. This is very different from your person passively submitting to treatment, and as a result, long-term success is much more likely.

⌒⌒

When approaching a conversation for the purpose of making an agreement, make sure you are clear—both for yourself and your person—about the purpose of the conversation. Openly invite the person's input and start a back-and-forth that can and will evolve over time. Conversations about agreements don't start with statements or opening gambits for give-and-take negotiations.

To invite someone into the conversation, it's key to clearly connect that conversation to a concrete decision. Relationships with people affected by SUD tend to have long histories, often tinged with conflict. Deliberately or incidentally, hiding the intent with vague and ill-defined invitations, such as "There's something I want to talk to you about," or worse, "We need to talk," can bring up all sorts of anxiety for your person.

Is this a big talk or a minor talk? Am I in trouble? If I accept, will I just be walking into judgment? Worries and assumptions about the matter of the talk create dread, and it's hard for anyone to enter a conversation open-mindedly in that headspace. Confusion breeds conflict, ambiguity activates anxiety, but clarity promotes kindness.

An invitation that has a clear context creates an entryway for open dialogue: "In family therapy last week, I noticed that you brought up your living situations. It sounds like coming home isn't a good option for you, and you really want to engage in more of a community living situation. Can we talk about the financial aspects of that?"

As this door is opened, having a script or endpoint in mind may be counterproductive. Agreements are not formed in single conversations—information and input must be gathered and considered. You may have come to this conversation with a proposal in mind, a certain percentage or dollar amount or duration of support you can afford to give to help them in their success. It's good to know those limits so you can feel secure in what you can offer—but that's not the purpose of the conversation.

When you invite your person's participation in the solution, you draw in *their* concerns and priorities as well. You need to gather their input as data so you can help them solve the problem, not impose a plan on their life. In response to this, they may say something like, "Yeah, the real problem is I'm going to need a reliable car."

You might not agree that the car should be the priority while they are in treatment, but arguing about how they define their needs is not productive. In that moment, the conversation's primary purpose is to gather information.

"Let's talk about how we can work this out," you might say. "What ideas do you have? Who else have you talked to about this?"

In asking questions, you'll better understand their perspective and needs, which will make your agreement stronger, no matter what form it takes.

If the agreement ends up being ineffective or unsustainable, it can be revisited in the same way you opened it in the first place. Agreements must be flexible because life has a way of stirring things up and refusing to comply neatly with well-laid plans. For instance, in an agreement over sharing a vehicle, circumstances may change or obstacles may become clearer as the agreements are put into practice. That agreement can be revisited in a new conversation. "Hey, is now a good time to talk about the car? I know we agreed to share based on this schedule, but it's not working out because now, on Tuesdays and Wednesdays, I'm left in a pinch without my car. What other solutions can we figure out?"

When agreements are developed between you over time, that mutual trust can grow and expand. You can become more actively supportive of your person's choices without sacrificing your wellness. In this trust, you can learn to be a clear-eyed advocate for your person, someone who knows their needs, their weaknesses, and their temptations. They know how to recognize thought patterns and honor boundaries *they* form in order to protect their gains in recovery. Every person is unique, so every path to recovery should be tailored. Clear-eyed advocacy is not about being on their side regardless of the behavior, nor is it about being the intermediary between the authority of treatment professionals and your person. Advocacy is about walking *beside* your person toward the recovery that works for them.

Of course, an agreement formed is not always an agreement kept. However, when agreements are made with a focus on *clarity* rather than *permanence,* it is possible to revisit the agreement and find a way forward. This, like all aspects of agreements, goes both ways.

In forming an agreement, you may find yourself feeling unsure. You might feel like you're living on the razor's edge of what you would be comfortable with and what feels sustainable to you, whether the agreement is about your support, your role in their treatment, or the frequency or form of visiting with each other.

Owning that discomfort and making a concrete plan for addressing it can help the agreement move forward.

For instance, you might say something like, "This is a little bit on the edge of what I'm comfortable with, but I'm willing to give it a try. Would you be open to trying and then revisiting this topic in a month?" Setting a specific date with a plan to revisit the question keeps expectations concrete and visible, even while maintaining the future flexibility of the agreement itself.

It's a good idea to follow through with agreements by putting the expectations in writing. This is not for the purpose of creating a static contract or giving either party a platform to punish the other if the agreement isn't kept. Instead, the purpose of your written notes is to keep a record of how the conversation went, what was decided, and why. If your person doesn't keep their side of the agreement, revisiting the conversation allows you to examine why that agreement isn't working.

Depending on the specifics of your relationship and your person's well-being, agreements may need to wait until your person enters treatment and shows their willingness to change. Otherwise, it's difficult to maintain any kind of open back-and-forth. Boundaries, because they are not collaborative, can be formed in any stage: active addiction, contemplation of recovery, treatment, or sobriety. When we attempt to make agreements before our person is truly willing and ready to participate in collaboration, the arrangement rarely works. In these cases, agreements may make it more difficult to maintain your boundaries and contribute to the cycle of negative behavior patterns.

But when you are both ready, agreements can be the foundation for lasting change and a new, sustainable way of being.

When our son moved to Utah, we collaborated on an agreement for how we could support and partner in his decisions in his new life. We agreed on a certain number of months that we would pay for his sober living center, and we set clear and explicit expectations around the support. We didn't just go with the flow of his decision, tossing money at him to ensure he wouldn't have to feel the blow of any possible consequences. We didn't rely on unspoken expectations with the hope that everything would turn out okay.

The agreement was a true agreement—a collaboration that considered everyone's needs and boundaries. The reality of the situation was that he was going to make his own choices as an adult. We could either show up and create parameters around what was going to work for us and what was not going to work for us, or we could fight and hang him out to dry.

There is a false and dangerous dichotomy that underlies many notions about the families' role in SUD recovery, and it showed up in the therapist from our son's former treatment center. Either our son would follow the plan we wrote for him, or he was certain to fail. From that viewpoint, giving our son support in his move to Utah was the equivalent of giving him more rope to hang himself with.

But this point of view dismisses any possibility that our son could truly regain agency and control over his own life in a healthy way. The truth is, if we had not had the runway of our Parallel Recovery, we likely would have provided more rope. But because we had been doing our job of identifying patterns and needs, working in small ways to communicate and engage differently, and setting smaller (hamburger) boundaries along the way, we walked next to him, successfully empowering him to step into his long-term recovery.

You are not "helping" them by governing their choices through rules, nor would you be "supporting" them by shielding them from any natural consequences of their behavior. Denying someone's autonomy stands in the way of their true and lasting recovery.

It is only through collaborative agreements that you can provide actionable support to your person's recovery, ensuring that they are driving the car of their own life.

Our son's move to Utah was successful because we worked *with* him to create the support he needed. We haven't looked back since. We've only moved forward.

CHAPTER 12

LABELS AND LANGUAGE

A COMMON QUESTION I'm asked about people I have worked with in recovery is, "How long have they been clean?"

My response is always the same. "They were never dirty," I tell them. "They have been *sober* for..."

The goal of my gentle correction is not to shame the person asking me the question, but to be a positive part of the cultural shift around the way we think and talk about these problems.

In the past few decades, there has been a shift in the words and labels we use to discuss SUD, people affected by SUD, and treatment. Change is hard. Old-school labels persist, even for those actively doing the work of recovery and the professionals who guide them. As awareness grows, there is sometimes a cultural clash over these words. People express frustration, arguing, "You know what I mean," and, "Those terms have worked for years just fine."

But have they worked? Or have people managed to recover *in spite of them?*

When people refer to themselves using these words, they have bought into the label that culture has assigned to them. Perhaps that label has worked for them, but what would happen if we could change the labels culturally? How much better and easier could it be to ask for and receive help if we could remove some of the cultural and psychological obstacles?

Part of our job as affected family members is to start changing those labels. By gently refusing to apply them, we can move the needle and begin to unwrite the cultural narratives that get in the way of recovery for all of us.

The guidelines around words and language in this chapter are not about creating rules so you can avoid some imaginary "PC police" or authority that will trigger consequences if you use the wrong terms.

Words and language are a core and essential part of how we form connections with each other as people, so the words we choose really do matter. Words carry with them so many layers of meaning and connotation. When we choose the words and labels we use for each other, we not only affect those attached to those labels; we also define the place they hold in *our* minds, which in turn shapes how we speak to and behave around those we want to connect with.

Dehumanizing language is a way to distance ourselves from particular "types" of people with particular life experiences. When we use these terms, we give ourselves permission to consider them fundamentally less than us. We wrongly put conditions on basic human dignity. Conversely, when we use conscientious and person-centered language, we center the *person* and not their behavior or experience in our minds. This supports our ability to love and connect with them where they are.

The need for conscientious language applies outside the context of substance use and addiction as well. Calling migrants "illegal aliens," for example, implies that these people are inhuman and immoral for existing in a particular place. The phrase deprives people of their humanity, robbing them of the dignity and respect that should be granted to all people.

Basic words like "addict" and "alcoholic" may simply seem like accurate descriptions given the patterns of their behavior, but they also relegate people into categories that deny the complexity of their human experience and make their value contingent on their behavior rather than on their humanity.

Words are more than their relatively static dictionary definitions; they carry with them connotations and shared cultural images that evolve over time. Associations accumulate in our shared understanding. Each cultural depiction of what an "addict" looks like contributes a layer that deepens that image, making our shared vision of what it means to be an "addict" entirely negative and behavior-centered.

The negativity surrounding that image has accumulatively grown so heavy, that when it is applied to a person, it has a way of pushing all other descriptors away. It carries with it an unspoken "just" so that the person becomes not only an addict but "just an addict." All other roles, traits, and points of connection are discarded, as though they no longer matter in the face of SUD.

Focusing on the problems created by our person's behavior distracts us from the basic and fundamental fact that they are a person. We, as humans, thrive on our connections with others. Each time we attach dehumanizing words to people in our lives, either aloud or in our minds, we make a little cut in our human connection to that person.

Changing the words we use changes the way we think, even if we aren't always aware of how deeply those biases and patterns of thought are rooted in our minds. And the way we understand a person in our minds guides how we interact with them.

The goal of boundaries and agreements covered in the previous two chapters is to put borders around yourself regarding behaviors so you can find ways to maintain your connection with the person you care about, separate from their condition and their behavior. When we refer to someone as "a person experiencing substance use disorder" or "a person experiencing alcoholism," we're not denying the person's choices. Rather, we acknowledge that these are dangerous and difficult experiences of a human, not inherent or inalienable defects.

Many people resist changing their language habits. Accepting that you should now alter the way you speak about and address people—both directly in your life and at a distance—carries with it feelings of guilt that you may have been unintentionally hurting people this whole time. No one wants to be "part of the problem," so it's instinctual to want to avoid that shame by denying the need to shift their words and usage.

Often, when people resist this type of change, they push it aside as unnecessary and shallow, like a window dressing around feelings rather than the feelings themselves. But if the actual, specific words we use really were inconsequential, then it wouldn't be difficult to change how we use them. The first step in Parallel Recovery is embracing the ways *we* can change as well, and that includes the way we speak.

That is not to say we must adopt a rigid lexicon or constantly police the way others speak, especially about themselves. But we can become aware of the power our words can have and deliberately decide to center the *person* in our communication.

Person-centered language emphasizes the humanity and dignity of individuals rather than defining them solely by their condition or their behavior. This fosters a supportive environment and makes people feel respected and understood.

There are measurable effects to using person-centered language. It's clear that it works when it comes to supporting people during treatment and keeping them engaged through the whole process.

This subtle language shift also helps families and providers. When we change the words we use, we don't just *perform* acceptance, support, and non-judgment but we give ourselves a basis for adopting those attitudes all the way down. We help families and providers see people holistically, consider their unique experiences, strengths, and needs, and act accordingly in our unspoken communication as well.

Over time, this shift can become just as accumulative as those negative connotations and spread to change the greater public perception. The negative layers of meaning that have built up around "addicts" can be shifted away from the individual people and onto the disorder, where it belongs.

Often, we tell ourselves, *Well, I'd never say that out loud,* but the things we think still come out, influencing how we speak and act. Even if we try our best to soften our words as we express them, when we try to control others' behavior with our language choices, that authoritative judgment still comes through in our communication.

In many ways, our culture is one that measures our value not by who we are, but by what we do, especially those things we do better than others. Judgment bombards us from all sides, sending constant messages about status, prestige, appearance, and productivity, which creates an environment that is difficult to thrive in. Reinforcing that judgment through our words and actions adds an additional layer to the internal belief that worth is based on what we do, not who we are.

When we put down our judgment, we can create lasting shifts in our perception and mindset.

~

Often, when I work with family members whose loved ones aren't ready or motivated to engage in recovery, one of my first pieces of advice feels counterintuitive: Stop talking about their drug use or drinking.

You might have clear eyes that their use or drinking is the root cause of many other problems. You might be able to see that their consumption has steadily increased over time until it's starting to affect their health. But if they don't see their use as a problem, your focus on their behavior only shifts their perspective away from the consequences they need to address.

Instead, talk about how they feel in the mornings. Ask questions about their other recently strained relationships. Invite them to share the problems that are coming up at work.

Engage them with genuine curiosity and invite them to connect with you.

Changing the focus to your connection can start shifting your mindset and help you strengthen that connection separate from the adversarial feelings around their behavior. Behavior and identity can become intertwined, but where behavior feels changeable, identity feels so much deeper. Identity feels permanent.

Some family members I work with feel compelled to sell me on their person. They talk them up, sharing that they are a good person at heart and they deserve a better life.

Of course they are, and of course they do. I don't need to be convinced; I understand that this behavior can be separated from who they are as a human being. Part of our work involves changing things like our language to ensure that this belief is being communicated to our person as well.

We are all capable of behavior that doesn't represent who we are and want to be. Fortunately, we are also all capable of change.

∿

Words can also serve as barriers for those who might seek timely help or treatment for SUD. Those cultural images of "addict" and "alcoholic" exist in their minds as well, and when that image does not resonate with their self-image, it can reinforce the idea that their use is fine and acceptable, even relatively harmless.

Our self-image is always more complex than a stereotype and more encompassing than our behavior from moment to moment. Most of us would admit that we have told lies at different times in our lives, but we would also firmly reject the label of "liar."

"Yeah, I drink, but I'm not an alcoholic."

"Yeah, I party, but I'm not a junkie."

We can hear these protests and disagree, but this creates conflict centered not only on what they are doing but also who they are. When we do this, we don't get through to them as a person—we simply butt heads with their SUD. From the position of adversary, we can neither recover from our trauma nor support their recovery.

Words that attach to the core person—addict, alcoholic, junkie, doper—ask people to alter their self-image in a way that slots them as fundamentally separate from others. Until they fit the cultural stereotype those words represent, they understandably reason that they must not be "bad enough" to need help. It's no wonder these words create conflict. *No one* wants to pin on a negative label.

For someone with SUD, their understanding of the line between what is "acceptable" use and what is a problem has a tendency to drift further and further away. My son shared with me some insights on how this experience felt for him. In his social circles, he was surrounded by others who were also "experimenting" with substances and drinking. He always felt sure that he knew where the uncrossable line was. He could tell himself, "Whoa, that's not me. I'm not going to cross that line," but he didn't recognize that for him, the line was defined by his self-image and not his behavior. So the line kept moving, with him always on the "right" side of it.

Then, one day, he reached everybody's finish line. The people he had been with had do-not-cross lines, too, but they were all now well behind him. SUD can do that; it can hide itself until it is deeply ingrained into the mind.

During this time, I was more focused on trying to control his behavior than connecting with him as a person. My fear was in control, and it shaped how I spoke to and treated him. He pushed back because the message I expressed to him didn't fit with how he saw himself. His focus became countering my labels rather than paying attention to what was really happening to him. This is why internalizing these labels often delays the start of treatment and makes it much more difficult for your person to willingly step into the treatment process.

When a person *does* recognize that they need help, those internalized labels still act as a barrier. These labels are associated with people no one wants to be around or even have in society. They have been downgraded, shunned from the community.

These associations lead people to isolate themselves because they have accepted themselves as unwanted. For anyone to start a long, difficult process for their own good, they first have to truly believe that they deserve better for themselves. Without true connections with others, people are left feeling unworthy of asking for what they need.

⌒

Language is continuously evolving, as is the work surrounding addressing SUD on an individual and societal scale. The more we learn about what is effective treatment, the more we learn that empathy is an essential element to reaching others. Empathy can be developed individually and can also be supported or harmed by the language we use as a society surrounding these issues. As family members and conscious members of our communities, it is important we do our best to be conscientious about our choices in language, even when we are faced with difficult distinctions.

A difficult dichotomy of language has surfaced in reaction to the growing concerns about fentanyl, an extremely powerful opioid. In recent years, fentanyl use has increased in extremely dangerous ways, including counterfeit pills and inconsistent amounts added to other illicit drugs, dramatically increasing both the addictive properties and the risk of overdose. This added factor has significantly increased the incidents of drug-related deaths among a wide range of socioeconomic backgrounds and communities.

In response to this very real and serious trend, there is a growing separation between the terms "fentanyl poisoning" and "fentanyl overdose." Fentanyl poisoning is generally used by families who have lost a loved one suddenly and unexpectedly to a fentanyl overdose, often when the substance of fentanyl was not sought or when it was mixed with another less imminently dangerous substance without the person's knowledge. Fentanyl overdose is generally used to describe the loss of a person with a known history of disordered substance use, either fentanyl itself or other illicit drugs that are increasingly commonly tainted with fentanyl, such as cocaine or heroin.

This is a complex and sensitive subject. While an entire chapter could be spent on this topic, I would like to invite you to consider the impact of the implicit separation of those who die by fentanyl and were not known to have a substance use disorder and those who die by fentanyl with a substance use disorder.

The distinction and distance created by the separation of these terms unintentionally perpetuates the belief that "addicts" are worse and less deserving of health and even life than others. It categorizes some as victims and others as people who made a choice and thus deserve to die. Ultimately, this separation prevents people from recognizing a problem and getting help that they both need and deserve. In consideration of the fact that the majority of fentanyl overdoses were unintended deaths as opposed to planned suicides, I have made a conscious decision in my work and relationships to use the terms "unintended overdose" or "died by fentanyl."

⌒

There is a pervasive myth in our culture: "Once an addict, always an addict." This is not true. Even more troubling, this myth works against recovery. According to SAMHSA research and their developing definition of recovery, 72 percent of people who have had

SUD consider themselves to be in recovery or recovered from their drug or alcohol use problem.

Substance use can have terrible consequences and health outcomes, which is, of course, why it is such a scary behavior to see in our loved ones. But the idea that there is a sudden "switch" in the brain that flicks and, from then on, the brain is eternally an "addict's" brain is false. Addiction is a sliding scale that can show up in various forms and levels of severity. The DSM-5 (Diagnostic and Statistical Manual of Mental Disorders, 5th edition) includes a scale of mild, moderate, and severe diagnostic criteria to address the idea that there is no switch; it's a spectrum that can increase if not treated. Full recovery is possible from any stage, but it is much more approachable when addressed early. Making the decision to get help early or in moderate stages of SUD is much more accessible to people when it doesn't require them to accept negative labels for themselves. Simply put, labels keep people sick.

When families work together toward recovery, it raises the chances for success even further. When families are engaged in a Parallel Recovery process, their loved ones have a 64 percent success rate in seeking reduced use or complete abstinence. The results continue to go up when the commitment is sustained. Families who engage in this support for a year or longer see an 82 percent success rate.

These higher success rates can also be seen with early engagement. Research shows that when a family engages in training, they are significantly more likely to engage resistant and unmotivated loved ones, encouraging them to participate in treatment and recovery. Simply put, walking alongside someone in recovery simply works better than trying to push them through it.

A big part of the training in programs like CRAFT (Community Reinforcement And Family Training) and Parallel Recovery is learning how to first change our internal labels, then more effectively communicate and connect with our person. The language we use is an essential tool in doing this work.

There is so much positive potential in the work of Parallel Recovery. Research clearly shows that people can recover from SUD and live the majority of their lives in healthy and fulfilling ways. My family and the families I work with bear this out as well —it's not easy, but it's very possible.

It may come as a surprise, then, that I do have some words of caution about another word I hear often in my practice. While many people believe this word is positive, I discourage families from using it, especially when they are just beginning their parallel journeys.

That word is "hope."

Hope can represent a wonderful thing—a belief in the possibility of a positive and better future for yourself. Hope can serve as the opposition to despair, which is the feeling that nothing you can do will ever matter.

But hope can also stand in the way of loving your person *right now*, exactly as they are, despite their behavior. Hope alludes to the need to change in order to be okay.

Hope is a positive *belief*, but as an *action*, it is not enough. If you could hope or pray this problem away, it would be already gone. If your hope is focused on bringing about a particular outcome for your person, it's likely to muddy your ability to accept the way things are *now*. Love your person the best way you can in this moment—not the future, unrealized moment you're hoping to manifest.

Hope for relief from the things you feel during the darkest times. Hope that you can take what you've learned and move forward in a better way. Hope that you can form a stronger connection to your person.

Don't direct your hope toward the day your person has changed, the day you can finally love them.

Love them now.

PART FOUR

GRIEF

CHAPTER 13

AMBIGUOUS GRIEF

BY THE TIME we are near adulthood, we expect to feel the acute and powerful sadness of loss from time to time. Our culture holds a space around loss, specifically, a space around the grief that follows a death. Even before we feel that grief, our culture tries to prepare us for it by surrounding it with reverence. We learn to pull over when we see a funeral procession. We refer to ourselves and others as "in mourning," as though the grieving have moved into a different place altogether, not in the world at all. Our cultural and familial practices teach us to grant patience, space, and support to those who have lost a loved one.

But grief is often more complicated than that. Grief doesn't have clear bookends. And it also doesn't require a well-defined loss or tragedy.

Ambiguous grief is a complex form of grief that is experienced without an actual death or loss in the traditional sense. Since the visible grief associated with mourning is accompanied by so many cultural traditions—traditions that only happen when an actual defined death or loss occurs—ambiguous grief can be enormously isolating. It can be as all-encompassing and painful as any other form of grief, but it lacks clear definition, causing those who experience it to question the validity of their feelings. Often, denial and dismissal of emotion follow.

The pain we feel when someone we love is affected by SUD is a form of ambiguous grief, and the first step to addressing it is giving it a name. Even when our loved one is still living, acknowledging and naming the loss we feel allows us to step into our recovery with willingness and understanding.

This experience hurts us because we love. It hurts us because we're scared. It hurts us because, while our person may not be gone, the way we feel and understand our relationship has significantly changed.

When we avoid these thoughts and deny our feelings, we naturally seek out coping mechanisms that represent the shadow side of our values rather than the best and most loving versions of ourselves. To maintain our denial, we try to manage unpleasant circumstances, believing that this will make the pain go away. If we can only change the external facts, then we think we can avoid the internal pain.

But this only puts off the hard feelings that we will eventually need to process. The hard-easy path starts with recognizing and naming what we are going through. Its name is grief.

When someone is grieving, there's no band-aid solution. The only way out is through. And that is the same with ambiguous grief.

One day, my son was leaving the house. A simple action, a tiny moment, but I remember it so clearly.

He was on his way out the door wearing shorts and flip-flops, despite the chilly February weather. It was during some of the worst times we experienced with his SUD. He was still living with us. Treatment had been attempted perhaps a dozen times, but he was still locked in active addiction. Everything in our home was friction, anger, and pain.

Now, someone was picking him up to take him God-knew-where. I stood there and watched him leave, desperate in my love and fear for him. He turned back to look at me, and there passed between us a moment of silent understanding.

Suddenly, everything seemed different. Before the door closed behind him, I had no idea that I had been existing in black and white. But when that door latched, my house—my home—was suddenly in full color. Everything was vivid and painfully clear. I'd been hearing sounds as though my ears were stuffed with cotton. As soon as he left, I could hear the neighborhood sounds in symphony.

The clarity overwhelmed me.

I had known for a while that this could be the last interaction that I would ever have with him. That every interaction could be our last. That he could die. I was desperately afraid of that possibility, not only for his sake, but because I feared what that would do to me.

The clarity I felt in that moment was different. I realized that, as I stood there, I was not proud of who I was in our relationship. I would be okay if he didn't come back. But I was not okay with what he saw, felt, and heard from me in those moments. He'd taken an experience of me out the door with him, and it was not the one I wanted him to have.

I stood there looking at the closed door, taking in all the colors and sounds. It lasted maybe two minutes, but it felt like two months. I was realizing my need to recognize who I had become. Somewhere along the line, I had been hijacked by the emotion, stress, and grief of the relationship. The world had to slow down to show that to me.

For me, that moment was the sign that *I* needed to change. I didn't know then exactly what that would look like, but it was clear that we needed something different.

So, I thought to myself, *what are you going to do?*

I had asked myself a version of that question a million times before—what are you going to do to help him? What are you going to do to get him to stay in treatment? What are you going to do to make sure he gets and stays healthy? What are you going to do to keep him alive?

In this new world, that question felt different.

Suddenly, the question was about me. What was I going to do to change how I was in this relationship? What internal work did I need to do to get and stay healthy? Because I wasn't healthy. And it was profoundly shaping the way I was showing up in the relationship.

I was so caught up in grief that I couldn't see who I had become. In all my striving to bring back the way things had been— the ways I had expected and wanted them to be—I'd lost sight of myself.

From then on, everything changed.

⋀⋀⋀

All forms of grief can come at us in waves.

If you've ever been in the ocean, you know how immutable waves are. They can't be stopped, redirected, or diminished. Waves gather force as they move through the water, and that force can carry you along with it. It can drag you under. But it doesn't have to.

To experience that wave in a way that keeps your head above the water, you have to respect its force. If the water is around your chest and belly and you dig your feet into the sand, you can tell yourself that you will not be moved, that you can keep yourself upright by sheer force of will. Telling yourself you will stay steady will not protect you. That wave is coming, and it will pull you in.

No matter how firmly you lock your muscles and insist that you are a pillar and that nothing could ever unseat you, that wave is coming. The water will crash into you, and that sand will be sucked out from under you. Up will turn to down and sky into foam.

But if you leave your feet loose and let yourself bob with the wave, letting its motion move you, it will set you back down where your feet can find the sand.

It's scary to let the wave carry you, even for a short time. It feels out of control. But the wave is more powerful than you are, and by respecting it, you can keep your head above water.

Grief works much the same. Ambiguous grief can knock us over even when we don't expect it. Since there's no clear beginning to ambiguous grief, it's impossible to anticipate and difficult to define. Recognizing it is the first step to navigating it differently. We can stop trying to dig our feet in the sand, denying the incoming wave, and feel what we are really experiencing. We can let go of trying to control the external facts.

Ambiguous grief doesn't always carry with it the suits and trappings of compassion from culture, but it is still something that requires self-compassion. Self-compassion is knowing that you can't stand in the wave without being moved.

When people return to use, it's one of the hardest points of recovery. Some people, including some treatment providers, treat "relapses" as if they automatically reset progress to square one. That can be devastating, but it's also not usually an accurate assessment for you or your person. For you, if you're also working through recovery and developing healthy skills, you can continue to practice those skills despite a setback. You can continue to model a better way of coexisting. And for your person, relapses don't have to send a person back into unwilling or unmotivated stages of addiction.

Such was the case with one family I worked with. The son had left a program that was working for him to return to use. In communicating with the family, I emphasized that we were not back at zero. This was hard, but we can weather hard things.

The son's SUD had garnered several consequences, including

legal and financial problems. The family had to process the emotional disappointment, and they also had several practical decisions to make. The challenge was in finding clarity between those two very different needs.

In order to navigate this new hurdle while maintaining their kindness and firm boundaries, the family had to revisit the skills they had learned through their recovery. While he had been in treatment, they had supported him practically with access to a bank account. The family had already decided that this was not a form of support they could continue in active use, but they wanted to maintain the connection and relationship they had built. The son had an upcoming court date, and they had to decide whether or not to attend.

Before they communicated with their son, I encouraged them to sit with their emotional experience and sort through things. Some of their feelings would be about them and their fear. Others would be about protecting their emotional, physical, and financial safety (boundaries). And, finally, some would be about inviting their son to continue their connection.

He didn't need them to be at the court date, and with the changes they needed to make around their financial and legal support, they knew that attending might muddy the waters. It was important that communication remain clear and unequivocal.

They realized that showing up wasn't really a way of supporting him; being there physically was more about their own needs. They wanted to see their son, even just to lay eyes on him. Acknowledging that this was *their* need didn't mean they shouldn't go. But they had to own their need *as their own* rather than putting that need on their son as an additional burden on him.

Clarity and intention are important pillars in maintaining a healthy connection at every stage of recovery. Understanding and acknowledging your emotional needs keeps you in control of setting your intention, communicating with clarity, and making thoughtful decisions.

But for this family, understanding which needs were their own was about more than just clear communication. It was also about allowing themselves to feel a need and responding to that need with self-compassion. Acknowledging that what they were going through was emotionally difficult allowed them to give the feeling the space it needed. In turn, they were able to communicate to their son that they would be present at the court date and that they would like to talk or connect over lunch if he was available and interested.

That invitation could be received very differently than communicating to their son that they needed to see and be with him and that they needed him to reciprocate.

They did not connect with their son that day, but soon, there were positive indications that their connection could be maintained and honored through this difficulty. He accepted and did not argue about the changes in financial support, and while he said no to lunch with them that day, he met with them on another day, one when he could meet with them on mutual terms. This wasn't the meeting they would have designed, and they still felt ambiguous grief for the way things could have been, but they accepted the reality of the situation in order to connect to their son as he was at that moment.

Ambiguous grief exists in formed families as well. When we marry someone, there is a clear and concrete expectation of what our future with that person will be like. Likely, you've spoken about it and made it a collective dream between you, imagining where you're going to live, whether you'll have kids, and how you will support each other. When that collective dream turns out to be very different from reality, it's natural to mourn that loss, even though what you're mourning is something you never really had.

When your partner struggles with SUD, it can be tempting to hold out hope for that unrealized life. Much of this urge grows out of fear for what life will look like. But that fear is often what stands in the way of recovery. Whether you stay or leave the relationship, the life you pictured is not going to manifest the way you pictured it. Even if your partner is able to seek treatment and work toward recovery, the original plan included someone who wasn't their best self. Going back there is not an option. That plan didn't include recovery. Your partner will be a different person, and life will need to honor that. Letting yourself grieve the life you'd dreamed of is the only honest path to making the decisions you'll need to make moving forward.

Working toward recovery may or may not look like working toward recovery together. I have worked with partners who have left a spouse in active use and who have watched as their ex-partners did, in fact, get better. Because they have worked through recovery skills themselves, they were able to love each other as separate co-parents and find positive ways forward in their new lives.

There's no Hallmark card for ambiguous grief. People don't set up meal trains because you're mourning a life that you wanted for someone else and are missing what you thought your life and theirs would look like. Still, this grief is a very real experience. We may all feel a need to minimize our experience, to pretend that our hearts aren't broken.

The waves of grief may come around would-be milestones. For me, the feeling of loss came the year my son would have graduated from college if all of my hopes and expectations for him had played out the way I'd imagined. Many family members describe being hit with these feelings around holidays or when they are returning to certain places that remind them of earlier and different times. These are the similar emotional triggers that people experience with "traditional" grief.

I hear people describe these feelings and then immediately try to diminish them—"Oh, that's just silly." The unspoken part of that dismissal is *at least they are alive.*

It's true that they are alive, and it's also true that ambiguous grief is a different experience from the grief that follows death. But ambiguous grief is still grief. You can show yourself compassion by giving it its name and allowing yourself to really experience what you're feeling. Ambiguous grief isn't selfishness or self-indulgence in not getting your way. The pain is real.

Imagine seeing an oncoming wave and saying, "Oh well, that's just silly."

Ambiguous grief doesn't have a silver lining. It's not "at least-ing" your experience. In itself, it is an experience that most of us would avoid if we could. If we could go back in time and unwrite the circumstances that created that pain, we would.

Toxic positivity asks you to be grateful for pain and to find a purpose in the pain. But often, that leads us to engage with our relationships in the hope that our person will show up differently. They will suddenly appear to make us feel better. Suddenly, we'll see that this was all worth it—it all happened for a reason.

Grief and hardship will come our way, and we can process them in a healthy way if we don't force ourselves to pretend they are good things.

People can become frozen in both grief and denial. Trapped in a constant cycle of fighting and pretending, we will reach for anything to get our heads above water. But if you allow the feeling to flow through and around you to a place of acceptance, you can eventually release the old image of your person in favor of the new one.

When we're missing someone, memories have a way of flashing upon us in clear and vivid detail: that smile or the warm sound of their voice or the shared look of common understanding or their love of hummingbirds. They are moments of awe we can remember, experiencing that which brought us joy in those moments.

Though grief and joy are strong feelings that are oppositional by nature, it is possible to experience them at the same time. Ambiguous grief may be such that you carry it with you nearly all the time, riding the bigger waves the best you can. The waves don't have to block those moments of awe, wonder, and joy in your life or even with your person as they are now. In fact, they may even raise you up to see those moments even more clearly.

We can have new moments of awe with our person. Things may look completely different—it may feel like a whole new relationship. But in the moments where you can find connection, you can still find love and joy.

CHAPTER 14

TRAGIC OPTIMISM

SUFFERING IS HEAVY. It can take up a huge space in our hearts and minds. We can't displace that weight—no one else can carry it for us. We also can't make it any lighter. Since it stems from the reality of our situation, no amount of sunny-side-up thinking can shrink it. But we can grow stronger and more resilient, making it easier to carry.

Hurt, like joy, can be found in a thousand little moments every day—even things as small and instant as a short text message.

Hey, happy birthday. I'm sorry I can't be there. I just can't.

In the greater context of life and relationships, this little message can be a lot of things. It can be a reminder of that painful, heavy weight when part of the reason they "just can't" is that SUD has strained the relationship. In the grand scheme of things, missing a birthday might not be a big deal, but in a larger, painful context, it's still a sharp sting.

Our desire for positivity may tell us to diminish the sting in our minds. We want to respond with *That's okay, no big deal.*

But talking about it as if it's nothing doesn't make it nothing. Rather, it adds a layer of unspoken resentment, invalidates our pain, and prevents us from processing our feelings. Conversely, it's also not helpful to take this moment as an opening to dig out further grievances and try to score points, as if there's some grand game to be won by having more scars than others. There's no scoreboard, and brewing conflict only deepens the hurt.

We don't have to hide from emotional difficulty, nor do we have to be a reactive victim to it.

I'm so sad that you can't be here. It just won't be good unless you can come.

This response expresses our pain, but it also adds guilt and burden to our person during a time when they are already struggling to show up.

Because how we feel is often complicated. We can feel hurt and joy in the same moment. We can acknowledge the grief and loss we're reminded of while still having a moment of gratitude for what we do have. It's hurtful that our person can't show up beyond a text message right now, but we can recognize they showed up the best they possibly could—by remembering our birthday and sending a text. We can feel and process both of those things and respond with intention.

Thank you for remembering me today. It means a lot to me.

Laid out in words as an example, it seems like such a tiny shift. But what the shift can represent is a deep change in how you view yourself, your circumstances, and your relationship to others. Our goal is connection, not connection on our terms. Intentionally finding value in each other and our surroundings is not the same as putting on a happy face or pretending the pain has a purpose.

We're not grateful *because* we got a text message that hurt us. It hurts that they can't show up better, *and* we can be grateful for the connection we do have. We don't have to pretend to shrink or celebrate our pains in order to treasure our joys.

Viktor Frankl, who we have referenced before, advocated for approaching life through "tragic optimism." This seeming oxymoron of philosophical attitudes first acknowledges that suffering is part of every human experience. It is not possible to coast through life experiencing only happiness and joy; pain and loss are inevitable. It is so inevitable that suffering is an inalienable part of the human experience that binds us all together. Suffering is not a weakness to overcome or a fault in moral character. It is human to want joy and ease, and it is the nature of existence to experience hardship, loss, and pain. Challenges are simply part of the deal.

As much as suffering is part of human life, so is growth. Frankl argued that even, or especially, in the face of hardship, human potential—the best possible versions of all of us—gives us an opportunity for learning and growth, for making changes for the better, and for imbuing our lives with meaning through intention and thoughtfulness. Remembering that there is always an opportunity to respond to challenges with intention can help us meet them face-to-face.

This ability to make choices through intention is powerful, and embracing it can make fundamental changes in how you experience your life as a whole, even though it cannot prevent suffering.

People can get lost in the idea that suffering is inevitable. If there's nothing you can do to lessen suffering, then why do anything? This feeling of helplessness is despair. Despair isn't feeling the reality of our suffering; it's making our experience of suffering worse by digging into it and losing sight of everything else. Our minds can grab hold of suffering and spin out, adding guilt and blame and anger, making everything worse than it really is. The reality might be genuinely awful, and there may be nothing we can do to reduce the suffering. But with mindfulness and intention, we can choose to see reality more clearly in its greater context and find ways to experience and even appreciate the good things.

If you're reading this, you likely have a loved one who suffers from SUD. That's your reality. It's painful for you to see and experience them in that condition. That is genuine pain, and it can be so heavy to carry and scary to face.

In our fear, our minds extrapolate to other thoughts. We try to place the root blame somewhere, filling us alternatively with guilt or anger. We try to find solutions in hopes that being the hero will make us feel better. We try to make the suffering make sense.

But these other narratives only converge to trap us in our minds until we can't see anything but the pain. And that is what brings us to despair—the moment we're blinded from everything but our own hurt.

Tragic optimism isn't about denying suffering or even conquering or overpowering it. Tragic optimism is about practicing mindfulness so we can stay aware of the greater context, which always includes ways forward, the possibility of positive future experiences, and the simple beauty of the world.

⌒⌒⌒

Practicing real gratitude takes time to build up, like a muscle, but you can start with simple techniques to shift your mindset and keep yourself centered.

Set aside a particular time of day to intentionally reflect on experiences you can be grateful for that day. It doesn't have to be grand: a particularly good cup of coffee or a satisfying lunch, a message from a friend that comforted you or made you laugh, a book you wanted being available at the library, a fresh-smelling breeze, a tall person helping you reach something at the grocery store, a moment of affection from a pet, or any number of beautiful little things you can experience in a day. When you deliberately reflect on these moments, you make the choice to hold gratitude in your heart; you decide to let it resonate rather than letting those moments pass you by without having an effect on your spirit. Setting this time as a practice can also train you to notice things like this throughout the day. If you know your intentional gratitude practice is coming, you'll find yourself more sensitive to those moments and more easily able to recognize and experience them as they come.

There are also meditative practices that can help ground and calm you enough to allow you to focus on those grateful moments. Breath awareness practice is taking time to be aware of your breath, taking slow and deep breaths, and focusing on the sensations of each inhale and exhale as you let other thoughts fall away.

Body scanning is taking time to mentally scan your body from crown to heel, noticing any areas of discomfort or tension. You can ease some tension in these moments by intentionally relaxing muscles that may be subconsciously held taut, but the purpose of this practice is not to make a list of ailments that need treatment— body scans are about making a deliberate connection with your body without judgment or analysis.

If stillness is difficult to maintain, mindful walking can also be a meditative practice. Leave your earbuds behind and take a walk while focusing on the sensations of the world around you. Feel the ground beneath your feet, the breeze on your skin, and the sights and sounds you encounter. In your mind, name and describe as many of those sensations as you can. More than "there is a breeze," note that the breeze is cool and bright and contrasts the warm soft- ness of the sunlight. Notice that the smell is well up into your sinuses with an almost minty sting.

The weather doesn't have to be picture-perfect for this practice —the earthy, dusty smell after a hard rain, the mouth-drying sharp- ness of winter air, and the heaviness of humidity are all worthy of notice and can help you reconnect to your senses and make you feel grounded in the moment. Listen carefully to the sounds of nature and community around you: the melody of birdsong, the busy hum of traffic, the wind in the trees. Take in the brilliant colors of hummingbird feathers and the refraction of sunlight in the sky and over water.

More than finding gratitude, which might be hard at times, you can consider these moments as practicing awe. Your ability to feel awe can be exercised and made more available to you through deliberate practice. The world is truly awesome in the original meaning of the word, and taking a moment to notice those things opens the door to feeling that awe more often.

You may be wondering how these little easy practices—gratitude lists, breathing, walks—are meant to help with the complex and difficult problem you're facing. You're right. They aren't going to solve that problem or fix everything. They aren't meant to.

Mindfulness practice is a tool to build emotional and mental resilience. Mental resilience is just like muscular resilience. Exercise doesn't make weights actually weigh less; it just helps the muscles carry them safely. When you're resilient in the face of difficulty, you can better carry the weight of it without being overcome or losing sight of what really matters. You can still move forward, not because you dodged the weight or left it behind, but because you became stronger underneath it.

When some people tell you to take a mindfulness walk, they'll pair it with a story about how when *they* were on *their* mindfulness walk, they suddenly got hit with their big idea for the solution, the ultimate hack that really will fix everything, as if a clear head paves the way for a panacea. The unspoken implication is that if you can't find a tangible result—some grand new "purpose" from the practice —you must be doing it wrong.

Maybe in these practices, you'll feel some lightning flashes—a helpful epiphany. Probably not. These practices are about creating more emotional space for us to breathe and appreciate our lives. It's a practice that works little by little, and it doesn't have a goalpost. Success in this is not weighed by some external measure of accomplishment that visibly offsets your struggles. But cumulatively, the internal positive effects can be powerful. They can fundamentally change how you experience your life just as it is.

These practices do have real physiological effects. As I

discussed in chapter two, SUD can take a two-for-one in the ways that stress and despair raise cortisol levels and cause real and chronic pain. These practices can help counter that. Gratitude and mindfulness practices have been shown to lower cortisol, improve sleep, support the immune system, lower blood pressure, and lessen the physical symptoms of anxiety. Many of the physiological benefits come from activating the parasympathetic nervous system, also known as the "rest and digest" part of your automatic nervous system. It works as a counterbalance to the sympathetic nervous system, where fight-or-flight lives.

When we are confronted by big and painful problems outside of our control, we can get stuck in a constant stress cycle with an overworked and constantly stimulated sympathetic nervous system. The sympathetic nervous system isn't the bad guy here—we need it to survive and care for ourselves and others around us. By returning intentionality into our daily lives, we can help our systems come back into a state of balance, which is better for our health. When our health is improved, we are better able to show up and help our loved ones in genuine and thoughtful ways.

As we improve our mental health and lives, we are modeling that possibility for real and lasting change for our struggling loved ones and our greater communities. This practice can help foster and nurture our connection to our loved ones. It can create a positive feedback loop, strengthening that bond. The modes of communication are improved, reducing conflict and improving mutual understanding.

That connection has been shown over and over again to be a real lifeline for people struggling to find their way back to themselves. It's not guaranteed, and bringing about an external outcome is not the primary reason to engage in the practice.

Beyond our connection to our loved ones, mindfulness practice can have a ripple effect in our communities. Genuine and healthy optimism (as opposed to forced positivity) can have a real influence on not only our loved ones but on everyone we have sustained contact with. Your resilience can model resilience for others. It can even become communal resilience.

Practicing mindfulness and intentionality increases our capacities for empathy and compassion, which in turn helps us treat others as human individuals rather than harmful and reductive labels and stereotypes. This empathetic treatment helps encourage people to make better choices for themselves, and it also helps our greater community embrace people as individuals. Communities built on mindfulness and compassion have more effective altruism and support.

There is a fine but crucial line between tragic optimism and toxic positivity. As Frankl wrote, "Life is never made unbearable by circumstances, but only by lack of meaning and purpose."[1] He wrote often about finding purpose in suffering and being ennobled, not degraded, by suffering. He indeed found a close connection to the trials we go through and the value in how this makes us stronger and wiser if we look for the meaning in our experiences.

With toxic positivity, this core concept is being twisted and misused in many ways, and the core principles of this idea are often somewhat lost in translation and commodification. Toxic positivity tells us that we must feel positive no matter what and at all times. Hearing people make statements like "Don't let it get to you," "I don't let negativity in," or "Positive vibes only in this space" can make anyone wonder what they must be doing wrong when they feel pain from their circumstances. Gilding hardship in a silver lining is not helpful.

These kinds of statements are a dismissive and invalidating response to people expressing their pain, *and that causes more mental suffering.* Overly simplistic mantras like "purpose in the pain" don't get to the heart of the philosophy. When positivity is reduced to this tin-can advice, it becomes impossible to actually exercise, which in turn causes feelings of self-doubt, guilt, and inad-

---

1.   Viktor Frankl, *Man's Search for Meaning* (Beacon press, 1946).

Experiencing suffering doesn't mean you're too weak to let it roll off your back or too lowly to rise above earthly concerns. It simply means you're going through the human experience, and it is hard.

When you make space for mindfulness and gratitude, it exists alongside the ambiguous grief you feel in your circumstances. Taking a walk for your mental health isn't an obligation for you to triumph over your negative feelings. Those waves of grief are still here and will take you up for a time now and then. It's okay to let it; it's okay not to be okay all the time. You will also feel sad, angry, and frustrated, and you can let yourself feel those emotions and let them run their course. In those times between, finding space for gratitude and intentionality returns the balance and reminds us that life isn't *all* grief and darkness, nor is it all joy and light.

Tragic optimism is choosing to make room for positive emotions. It is not a cultivated blindness to suffering; it is a vote for awe.

Toxic positivity also tells you that what doesn't kill you makes you stronger, so you should be grateful for everything that doesn't kill you. This is absurd. It's no wonder people cannot live up to that standard. I've learned and grown a great deal in the past decade, but I do not thank the fire for taking my home.

Gratitude is a big part of how we can experience tragic optimism, but it is misplaced if you are asked to be grateful for what is causing you pain. Tragic optimism doesn't require you to perform mental gymnastics or to accept inherent contradictions. It's about stepping back to check in with the things we feel full-throated and honest gratitude for. It's not about diminishing suffering but rather about creating space for both joy and pain to exist together. That is much more sustainable over the course of a lifetime because it is authentic.

Toxic positivity can also be used as a shield. It hurts to hear that we might be part of people's suffering, especially when we hope for exactly the opposite. Pushing away that hurt with toxic positivity means rejecting the opportunity to find meaning, intention, and growth in that challenge. It pushes the responsibility away from yourself and onto others, prioritizing comfort over growth.

Many cite Frankl even as they deliver messages of toxic positivity. But it is not the pain itself that has a purpose. The purpose lives in you and how you choose to respond to painful circumstances. The meaning in our challenges is not a gift we receive from the universe or something we can accept passively. Imbuing our lives and experiences with meaning is an intentional and active choice.

The pain is just a fact. The purpose lives in you.

CHAPTER 15

RADICAL ACCEPTANCE

IT'S hard to hold space in your mind and heart for both grief and optimism. Especially when, for a long time, you've been trying everything you can think of to bring about a better set of circumstances for yourself and your loved one. I understand it may seem frustratingly abstract and even contradictory. When looking for a new strategy, it's understandable to want a clear path with concrete steps, measurable benchmarks, decision trees, and instructions.

But this isn't about how to have a new strategy. Strategies are about gaming circumstances in order to achieve a specific goal. Goals are good things to have, and working toward progress is healthy and commendable. But goals hyper-focused on an outcome can also carry with them dangers and blinders that keep us from appreciating and understanding our current circumstances.

You may not realize how *specific* your goals are in times of stress and dysfunction, but often, we carry with us a specific image of what it means to be "okay" for us and our loved ones. That image can keep us holding our breath, feeling as though as long as we put our heads down and push forward, we'll reach that finish line of "okay," and we'll be able to let go of our struggle and breathe easy again.

When your head is down, you can't really see what's around you and where you are going. Sometimes, what we really need to let go of is that specific goal of what "okay" means in order to bring our perception and emotional life in tune with the reality around us. Before we can work toward any progress, we should first understand where we are, even and especially if it's not where we want to be.

〜

Our connections to our loved ones and our communities are essential to our emotional lives as humans, but they can become so entangled that they start to blur the boundaries between our individual lives, needs, and perceptions.

In parental relationships especially, there is a cultural expectation that our happiness is contingent on our children's well-being, happiness, and even the fulfillment of *our* expectations for them. There is a phrase that circulates in the culture that may seem well-meaning but, upon closer inspection, has chilling implications.

You're only as happy as your saddest child.

This is intended to be a reminder of how deep a parent's love runs. It's true that a child's pain and suffering will always be difficult for a loving parent. But there is another layer of implication here, which indicates that a sense of peace or well-being is out of reach for any parent who has a child that is not currently experiencing peace or well-being. This way of looking at familial love keeps families trapped in a cycle of continuously compounding each other's pain through emotional enmeshment. The message is "I need you to be okay so I can be okay."

Emotional enmeshment is a psychological state where your emotional balance and well-being are so intertwined with the status of another person that you lose all sense of autonomy or separation.

Enmeshment is not the same as attachment or love; it is an unhealthy level of emotional entanglement that hurts both you and your loved one. A clear sense of self and individuality is essential for mental health and clear decision-making. Emotional enmeshment with a person who is suffering keeps us locked in a constant state of reactivity. We are always reacting to what they have done and what they need. Emotional enmeshment interferes with your sense of self and puts blinders on your ability to perceive the whole of reality around you, including your own reasons and the emotions behind your choices.

When you are emotionally enmeshed with someone who is not healthy, you are adding additional burdens to you both. For yourself, you are hurting your mental health and well-being by denying yourself space to feel positive things unattached to the well-being of your person. And for them, you are adding the burden of responsibility for your well-being on top of their own sickness and suffering. Sometimes, it doesn't feel that our person affected by SUD is aware of their behavior and well-being's effect on us, but they can feel that burden, and it does cause additional weight.

I have had a parent express to me their intense feeling of needing their child to be successful in treatment by saying that they would be "going down with the ship" if it didn't work the way she felt she needed it to.

SUD can indeed seem like being on a sinking ship; the disorder can be overwhelming, and the longer a person suffers from it, the less able they are to manage. Their "ship," so to speak, can become unseaworthy, and it takes enormous mental, emotional, and often physical effort to break free of that sinking ship and make treatment successful and sustainable. People can do it and *are* doing it every day, but recovery from SUD is a journey against the current. Would you want to add to that struggle the knowledge that they are carrying your well-being too? It certainly wouldn't help them swim.

You can't go down with the ship. That is not a viable path toward health for anyone. This trap of emotional enmeshment is why it is so important for families to work toward recovery alongside each other, addressing their own emotional needs and health in order to create an environment where true, individual recovery is possible.

It can be very difficult to recognize and untangle emotional enmeshment in families affected by SUD because of the uncertainty surrounding the future. The possibility of recovery is very real, but that vision of a recovered future becomes entwined with the relationship. The love felt in that relationship becomes dependent on that unrealized future. This tangle gets in the way of understanding and accepting the reality of the current situation, which in turn complicates that very path to recovery.

In a very different sense, there is a particular kind of grief surrounding a diagnosis of terminal illness and the families affected by such a loss. From the point of diagnosis, there is an understanding that the time available to spend together with your loved one is uncertain but very limited, and likely, that time is going to be marked with discomfort as your loved one's illness worsens and degrades the quality of their life. This is, of course, a very painful time, but there is also a natural progression that occurs as families grieve alongside the loved one's remaining time.

For the families, there is the future reality of when the person is gone and the reality of now when the person is still here. While it's natural for some to struggle to accept this, eventually, there is an understanding in this situation that there is nothing to be done but appreciate whatever time and moments of connection can be had. Though it is painful, families will often avoid adding to the burden and fear of the sick as much as they can. Every good moment becomes precious because they are finite.

The ambiguous grief surrounding families affected by SUD is very different in that the reality of now is not clarified by the knowledge of what is to come but muddied by what might be or might have been. There is no clear beginning nor end to SUD; the grief families feel is equally nebulous. This stands in the way of the important experiences that can be felt in the reality of *now* as it is and appreciating whatever time and moments of connection can be had.

There is an understandable instinct to do as much as possible as quickly as possible to prevent the worst possible outcomes. That instinct leads us to put all the focus and pressure of our efforts outward, but as we have learned, our attempts to control others simply will not work. We can only be in the driver's seat of our own life, and if we are putting all our energies into changing the external reality, then fear and pain control and drive our lives.

We know that SUD does not have to be a terminal diagnosis, but that doesn't mean we can't treat all the good moments as precious and finite now. We can still feel the reality of where we all are and accept the pain that comes from that situation as part of our life experience. By doing so, we won't miss our opportunities for real moments of connection with our loved one in our current reality. Your pain, all of a sudden, has the power to make those moments important and your connection felt and heard. This is where your influence lies. Otherwise, you just pass it right by because you're stuck in the reactive mindset of being a victim of what's happening to you.

Thus, the opposite of emotional enmeshment is not detachment but *radical acceptance.*

Radical acceptance is accepting the reality of what is true in the present moment without trying to will it to be different, denying its weight and meaning, or twisting it through magical thinking and wishful interpretation. When we embrace radical acceptance, it comes with accepting the painful parts of the way things are as part of the package. But it also embraces the possibility of all the positive and beautiful parts of the way things are. When you are engaged in trying to fight, control, or constantly reinterpret reality, your whole experience is tied up in that endeavor, and you miss the things that are in front of you.

Accepting reality doesn't mean you agree with it. It's not

saying, "This is fine because this is how it has to be." Nor is it throwing up your hands and resigning to total inaction and despair in its face. It's not saying, "I can do nothing to change this, so I give up."

To make strong and healthy decisions, we have to see reality clearly. Much of the other emotional work I have described in previous chapters is reliant on clear eyes and intention. Our ability to take advantage of the pause—the space between stimulus and our reaction—is dependent on being able to take in and feel a greater context than just that singular stimulus.

Emotional enmeshment means that the only stimulus we are really paying attention to is the emotions and status of our loved one, so that makes it very hard to slow down and take that important pause. Being able to live true to our values and not the shadow sides of our values also requires that we are fully cognizant of ourselves as we are. When we are emotionally enmeshed, our sense of self is clouded, and we can't see the difference between our values and their shadows.

This work of recovery is full of hard calls and challenges, and we can only meet them with intention, love, and the best of our ability when we see reality clearly.

There is nothing easy about grief in whatever form it takes, but denying reality only makes it harder in the long run. Accepting the situation is the hard step toward finding an easier peace. Fear and pain can stand in the way of your intentionality. They can't be deleted or shoved aside, but they can be addressed. The hard-easy path toward recovery is accepting the reality of each day as it comes.

⁓⁓

Radical acceptance does not mean that you give up on forming and working toward goals, but it is not a tool to accomplish a specific task. It is a way of shifting your perspective and mindset so you can make realistic progress throughout your recovery and support theirs in the best ways you can, given their current needs and situation.

Depending on the nature and specific context of an individual's SUD, treatment plans vary widely. Some of the options available for treatment carry with them degrees of controversy, including different methods of harm reduction practices. Harm reduction meets resistance because it often doesn't fit the image people carry of what being better looks like, and some argue that it is simply exchanging one problem for another. Radical acceptance means that we don't have to embrace the methods as an ideal situation or end result but as a realistic step to take in order to reduce suffering and risk right now in the immediate reality.

Suboxone, for example, is a prescription medication used to treat opioid use disorder specifically. A person taking Suboxone as part of a treatment plan will "fail" a standard drug test, barring them from many jobs. It also disqualifies a person from certain treatment facilities who will not or are ill-equipped to monitor that use as part of a comprehensive program. Certain medical treatments also may be complicated or made impossible while taking Suboxone. It is a serious substance, so dependence and withdrawal are still concerns, and it should be carefully monitored throughout its use.

In short, no one looks at being on Suboxone as an ideal healthy lifestyle one should aim for. No one starts off picturing their child, partner, or loved one someday on this difficult medication for any amount of time, and it can be difficult to accept it as a viable option toward health. But no one considers chemotherapy to be something they'd "opt in" for either. The reality is that sometimes it's necessary. Sometimes, it's the only step forward.

For someone in active opioid addiction, especially those nearing a crisis point, Suboxone is a route toward a significantly improved quality of life and reduced risk of overdose and permanent physical damage. In many cases, Suboxone can work as a rounded path toward living without reliance on a substance. It's not a straight line, but sometimes recovery simply cannot take what feels like the shortest and most direct path between two points. Just because you can imagine a specific, better set of circumstances doesn't mean you can force them by jumping straight there. The long way around is still progress, and it can still be appreciated for every measure of increased safety, health, and connection. But not without radical acceptance.

Also, imagined circumstances and specific goalposts exist for you in a way that may not for anyone else, including your loved one. When we are emotionally enmeshed, it can be difficult to recognize when we are imposing goals rather than supporting progress. When we've spent enormous time and energy trying to persuade our loved one to seek treatment and to see how much better things can get after SUD, it's tempting to keep going and pushing towards other goalposts that may or may not be part of our loved one's healthy life or definition of what it means to be "okay."

A common goal for parents when their children are on the path of recovery is to get them back into college and on the track we expected. In a conversation about a young man in recovery, his parent expressed to me that "I just want him to go back to school." I invited her to really play back what she had just said. After doing so, she amended that, "He really wants to go back to school too."

That very well may be true. But he also knows that *she* wants him to go back to school, and that has a big influence on his thinking. Along the line, part of her specific image of what "okay" means came to include not only health and safety but being on a particular path.

Working on recovery takes a lot of mental and emotional energy, and all his internal resources may be needed in order to make that sustainable, especially in the early months. Going back to school would add a significant amount of stress, pressure, and responsibility to that already pretty full plate. Not to mention that college, for many young people, is where SUD really takes root, so returning will likely involve a lot of emotions that could trigger intense desires to return to use.

The reality is likely that he is not in a place where a return to school would be successful. An unsuccessful return could be a costly and stressful mistake and a major step backward, not forward.

That doesn't mean he won't ever be ready. It may require a circuitous route to return to higher education or the kind of job path you may have always pictured for them. Or it may mean that the route forward takes them somewhere else entirely—not what you pictured, but better than where they had been and of their own making.

Radical acceptance is taking a frank and honest look at our true circumstances so we can understand what steps forward are genuinely available, which can mean letting go of that picture we held in our minds as "better." The truth is that there are many ways to be okay. The clearer we can see that truth, the wiser decisions we can make for ourselves and in supporting our loved one's decisions.

Radical acceptance doesn't stop even as things progress toward better circumstances.

There was a time when my son, in recovery, was between jobs and came back home for a couple of months. Having him home was wonderful and a challenge because it gave us a lot of time to connect, but we also all had more work to do on our recovery journey.

For over two months, he stayed in our guest room and spent his days working on customizing a 2000 Dodge police transport van. The project allowed him to spend time working alongside his dad, and this time of connection was invaluable. His vision for the end result was a true residence on wheels. Each day of work presented a problem to be solved, and over time, the plan was adjusted to fit what was possible with the time, energy, and money he had to put into it.

After two months, the result was something closer to a camper than the original livable home he had imagined, but that didn't mar his pride and love for what he had created. He was accepting the reality as it presented itself each day and appreciating each part of it that was good, which gave him quite a bit to appreciate, both in the process and in the result.

I wanted to support this project in every way that I could, but that took some adjustment on my part as well. As a naturally task-minded and energetic person, many mornings I would ask him what was on his list for the day and what his plans were. Finally, he turned to me and was able to express that this wasn't the best way I could support him. He shared that when I asked him these questions, it felt to him that I was discounting and invalidating everything he had done the day before.

I listened to this carefully, trying to take in that 10,000-foot view. It wasn't my intention to make him feel that way, and it didn't reflect what I wanted to share with him. To be better in my support, I had to accept the reality that my son's pace and style were simply different than mine. I had to adjust my approach to his pace if I wanted to really support him and connect with him in a way that could be heard and felt.

My family's reality and circumstances have changed in massive, impossible-to-miss, blessedly better ways in the past few years. But the work of radical acceptance continues as we adjust our plans to meet the real needs of the moment and appreciate everything we can about the journey.

PART FIVE

SELF-COMPASSION

CHAPTER 16

SELF-JUDGMENT VS. SELF-COMPASSION

WHEN WE SHARE the burden of change and reflect on our role in our relationships with our loved ones, we start to see our mistakes. There are two reactionary responses to this that are both understandable and unhelpful. Our minds will pick at problems looking for root causes. We want to find the moment things went wrong and assign blame to someone or something. We attach judgment to the way things are, and sometimes that judgment includes ourselves.

Blame and judgment aren't useful. There is no exact start or end point, so looking for root blame is a fruitless effort. Attaching judgment speaks of a finality that gets in the way of growth and change. Facilitating change requires compassion, and this includes the changes we can make for ourselves and our mental well-being.

When someone we care about is experiencing grief or going through a hard set of circumstances, we instinctively treat them gently, with extra kindness and patience. If someone you cared about was going through what you are right now, how would you approach them? You wouldn't expect to make the hard stuff stop—but you might ask them what they need and give them the support required to make it through that day. The help is in the space we hold for them, not in the act of removing their difficult situation.

Self-compassion works the same way. We can acknowledge how hard and painful our circumstances are and grant ourselves the same grace and patience we would a dear friend. What you're experiencing should not isolate you but rather help you find common humanity with others.

Compassion for others and compassion for yourself both start from a place of understanding.

In order to be a positive influence on our loved ones with SUD, we must first acknowledge that their behavior makes sense to them in the moment, in the same way our behavior makes sense to us in the moment. We might realize the next moment, the next hour, the next day, or even a year later that there was a better choice or a better way to show up in a relationship or situation. But realizing there was a better choice is only a single step toward being able to choose better in the future.

To understand, we can ask ourselves compassionate questions to try to find and understand our root needs. Your root needs are not faults, so we are not attaching blame but seeking a broader understanding of ourselves. Everyone has emotional needs, so needs are not holes in your character or weaknesses in your nature. When we react based on our emotional pain in the moment, the relief is fleeting and carries with it more consequences than benefits. We can't get rid of the need, but we can use time, reflection, and understanding to respond in ways to have that need met. And, most importantly, we can forgive ourselves for the mistakes we made before that time and reflection.

⁂

Self-care is important and can mean a lot of different things. "Self-care" has become a cultural buzzword that carries with it associations that can look superficially the same as self-indulgence.

But self-care is much larger than this. It includes the practical and concrete actions you're taking to identify and meet your needs. Self-care, in the literal sense of caring for yourself, is essential. The truth of "you cannot pour from an empty cup" is self-evident. What will genuinely keep your cup full takes a bit more to understand, and it might look different for each of us.

You're probably familiar with the imagery of #selfcare on Instagram and other social media platforms. There are always new lists of suggestions from skin and hair routines, cozy spaces to read, pretty habit trackers, healthy and interesting meals, time spent in nature, and so on.

These are all good things, and our self-care may include some of these aesthetic practices. Or it might not. It can be tempting for some to skip right into those things as actionable distractions from pain and discomfort. For others, it may seem impossible to imagine how any number of lattes or even good nights of sleep could possibly help. This is partly because the action of self-care is only a small part of what is really needed.

We also need the larger work of self-compassion.

Self-compassion is the internal work of naming, understanding, and intentionally serving your deeper needs. Self-compassion isn't dependent on external circumstances, which are fleeting. It's always available because it's an internal resource. When you develop high self-compassion, you are actually building greater resilience, which is the improved ability to withstand the difficulty of your circumstances. You can develop a better tolerance of discomfort because you understand how to self-soothe while also acknowledging what's happening.

Self-care can include helpful and healthful actions that can support self-compassion, but trying to skip straight to Instagrammable self-care actions often backfires. We slide into self-indulgence or avoidance. The feeling of being soothed is fleeting, if felt at all.

In that way, actions that may seem like "self-care" can be little more than band-aids to the greater problem. These can, in fact, be very much like using drugs or drinking alcohol—just a way to ease the discomfort of the moment. Even if those band-aids don't carry the same deep consequences as other coping mechanisms do, they often aren't whole or lasting solutions and can put off the harder and more permanent steps of self-compassion and self-forgiveness.

The compassionate question we should ask ourselves is not, "How can I make this pain go away?" but rather, "How do I name what it is and genuinely offer myself what I need for enough relief to move forward?"

There are practical tools that can be used to help you find that relief and strength to move forward: taking walks, mindfulness practice, taking time for your personal hygiene and presentation so you feel more like yourself, and letting non-urgent things go in order to give yourself space for rest and stillness. These are all positive acts of self-care. Their positive effects last longer when you understand *why* you are doing them and what needs you are soothing.

Self-compassion goes further because it makes these steps more effective and sustainable in the long term. Take, for example, the self-care action of saying no to a non-urgent obligation—think volunteering for your PTA's bake sale or serving on the board of your local museum. You may feel a sense of immediate relief from having one less thing to worry about with everything you have on your plate right now. Self-compassion is also understanding your limits and forgiving yourself for those limits right now. You deserve radical acceptance, too, after all. It is understandable that you feel resentment about giving more of your energy. Your energy is being eaten up with the experience of SUD in your family.

It may be an important part of your values and how you see yourself as the type of person who is helpful in the community and shows up for events like this. If this self-care action comes with later guilt and injuries to your self-esteem, then we're missing the bigger self-compassion step. Understanding that this is the limit you need to honor now in your given circumstances doesn't mean it will be your limit forever. Nor is it an indelible mark against your character. It's not weakness but preserving our strength for the things that matter and may be more urgent right now.

Self-compassion also recognizes that you're not going to be perfect. If you're showing up in a way that doesn't represent yourself accurately or effectively, self-compassion guides you to ask gentle questions of yourself to figure out *why,* so you can address those needs differently.

For instance, addressing our limitations informs how we communicate with people we care about.

Perhaps you are witnessing a person you care about rack up debt, fail to pay taxes, or keep a stable living situation because of financial choices. You may even be able to see from your perspective that SUD is behind a lot of these poor financial choices. They come to you to complain about these circumstances, which always escalates into an argument. You might lose your cool and communicate in harsh, unhelpful ways.

To figure out why you're not showing up the way you want to, you need to ask yourself why this bothers you so much and what it is you need in order to move forward in a better way.

You may have a core value around being a sensible and responsible provider for your household. Dependability and safety are crucially important to you and are tied to your self-worth. When you discuss the financial choices they are making—very different choices than you would make—you may find that it strains your ability to communicate with kindness and understanding. This makes sense since their actions are so against who you are and the way you live. Continuing a pattern of conversations that escalate into sharp words or raised voices is neither going to convince your person to change their behavior nor help you regulate your reaction.

Putting a boundary around discussing this topic is understanding and accepting your limits. It also communicates to your person that this is something core to who you are, that you've thought deeply about, and make careful decisions about every day. It may be counterintuitive, but this boundary can also serve as an invitation. Your person will remember that you communicated openly with them, and perhaps they may ask for advice at a later time when you are both ready to revisit the topic with grace. When your person considers making changes, they will remember that you are someone who takes this value very seriously. They may even see you as a source of wisdom once they are truly ready for advice.

Our limits now may not be our limits forever, but recognizing them in ourselves and in others is central to compassionate decision-making.

Holidays and vacations are cultural touchstones writ large on our personal and shared identities. When we tell ourselves the narratives of our lives, holidays and vacations stand out bigger and brighter than other days because of their imbued specialness. That importance is often due to the time we dedicate to spend together, celebrating our connections with one another.

While it's good to mark our years with special occasions, it can also come at a pressure cost that needs to be mitigated with grace.

Our connections to each other are deeply connected to our core human needs, and in our memories of how these connections are honored, holidays and vacations are big moments. This means that we want to recreate those times to re-experience the connection at the heart of those times. In our desire to recreate those holidays, the surface-level, material trappings of celebration can become our focus. Pressure can build as we struggle to plan just the right meal, convince everyone to attend and participate, hang the right décor, and honor all the traditions (with all the planning, accessories, and unseen work around those traditions).

This additional pressure can put everyone on edge, making it harder to feel a genuine connection. It's also worth noting that many of the traditions and events surrounding the holidays are intertwined with alcohol consumption, which complicates supporting a person in SUD recovery during these events.

The most compassionate thing we can do for ourselves and our families is to let go of our perfectionism and mental images associated with holidays and focus on how we may be able to connect in a mindful and supportive way for everyone. The elaborate meal with coordinated dishware and the Norman Rockwell picture may all be lovely, but it's not the actual reason holidays hold an important place in our year.

Letting go of those expectations can be wonderfully freeing. Tinsel, coordinated sweaters, and homemade, individual pumpkin pies aren't required to enjoy connecting with the people you love. Self-compassion can help you hear your need for celebration and connection and let go of the stress of creating a perfect picture.

Open communication in the time leading up to gatherings around the holidays may bring up some uncomfortable things, but addressing these issues ahead of time is the hard-easy choice, because diffusing tension in the moment is always harder in the long run. Discussing and creating safe and supportive spaces with clear boundaries ahead of time may be met with some resistance, but it is an important step. For example, you might ask family members to avoid certain topics of discussion that are no-gos or trigger points for contention. You might coordinate alternative activities to traditions that involved alcohol or took place in a certain home.

These conversations are not always easy or pleasant. Some may feel defensive about requests to accommodate others or about their own relationship with alcohol around these traditions. Beginning with your intentions for the boundaries can help everyone understand, if not agree. "It is important for me to have everyone together for dinner this year. I understand that we all have some reservations, so I am going to lay out a few off-the-table topics, so we all have the chance to enjoy dinner." Though uncomfortable, having these conversations won't take the magic out of the holidays. Rather, they will lay the groundwork of communication around what is needed for everyone to exist together in a safe space and enjoy being together.

The requests may not (probably won't) always be honored perfectly. The groundwork of communication allows for ways to more easily shift gears away from negative interactions. When you let go of the "picture" of that perfect holiday with self-compassion, it also becomes easier to be compassionate for others.

Self-compassion should not be confused with self-esteem. Self-esteem involves comparison, measuring yourself against others, your goals, and external societal standards. Raising your self-esteem often involves acknowledging things you've done well and setting reasonable goals. The inherent logic of self-esteem is reminding yourself that you completed X well once, which means you can do X well again and probably do Y well too. Celebrating your successes and setting goals is all well and good, but it might not be what is *most* needed in recovery.

High self-esteem can be useful in some circumstances, but it is fragile, dependent on those circumstances, and not particularly good at letting go of mistakes or overcoming internal obstacles. The inherent logic of self-esteem is all too easily applied to mistakes: You made A mistake, which means you will probably make A mistake again and probably B mistake too. That self-talk is reliant on comparison and judgment. It is defeating and *reinforces* your limits rather than accommodating them in the moment.

Self-compassion is taking time to reflect and explore your impulses, thoughts, and actions in order to discover your needs and limits. When you acknowledge and name the things you are experiencing today, you can think of how to find enough relief to keep going and show up even when things are heavy and hard. If you made a mistake, self-esteem would take that as evidence of who you are, the same as it would assimilate a victory. Self-compassion takes mistakes as evidence of what you are experiencing and how you are reacting to it. That exploration and self-forgiveness for that behavior is what is needed to prepare you for the next day of your experience. Self-compassion doesn't prevent you from ever making the same or similar mistakes again, but it does make room for better choices. It builds resilience in the face of those experiences and teaches you the habit of self-awareness.

Because self-compassion is not dependent on comparison, it also opens you up to being genuinely happy for others. Comparison leads to feelings of isolation—seeing people in similar situations find joy and happiness that feels out of reach to us in the moment can make us wonder what is wrong with us. When you let go of comparison in favor of self-compassion, you can find empathy and connection for others, even in their joys. Honestly honoring others' joys contributes then to your feelings of awe in the world, as you are identifying experiences that are wonderful instead of judging experiences that are better or worse than your own or others.

You are not alone in your experiences, and this struggle should not isolate you. Everyone's path to recovery may look a bit different because there is no real straight line to recovery, nor is there a singular destination or end point. Though we may not take all the same steps, we are not walking alone.

No one outgrows the need for self-compassion. We don't stop making mistakes or experiencing hard things or having needs. But we can get better, stronger, more resilient, and healthier than we have been.

Self-compassion is a fundamental tool in facilitating that change, and when we are able to show that growth and make different choices ourselves, we also become models for making that change for others. We can learn to name our experiences, understand our reactions, and choose ways to weather the difficulty in a way that can be more helpful than the ways we've chosen before.

Recovery from SUD requires that individuals learn to feel their need to self-soothe through substance use, understand why that need is there, and choose differently. Self-compassion is as essential in that recovery process as it is in ours, so in practicing self-compassion, we are also modeling the very human potential for change and growth.

CHAPTER 17

U-TURNS

MANY ADDICTION TREATMENT professionals evaluate individuals in recovery according to a clear and incremental set of "stages." The approach is deceptively linear: precontemplation, contemplation, preparation, action, maintenance, and, sometimes, return to use or "relapse."

There is an intertwined set of hopes and fears around these "stages" held by many families who watch the people they love go through them. Many hope that if they can only facilitate and convince their loved one through the action stage, then their "recovery" will have started, and their part is done. There is also a fear that any mental or emotional wavering in their loved ones in later steps will bring about the dreaded reset to one.

When families begin work on their recoveries parallel to their loved ones, they sometimes carry that same two-sided coin of hope and fear into the process. They hope that once they get to a certain stage, they'll have a clear action plan, complete with comprehensive and concrete dialogue trees and flowcharts for all contingencies and scenarios. They fear that if they falter along the way, all the work of reflection and soul-searching and trying to be better for ourselves and those we love will have come to nothing.

This sort of mental rigidity—sometimes thought of as "discipline"—is unrealistic and unsustainable. This all-or-nothing belief is not always articulated but sometimes comes out in the ways we judge ourselves and our loved ones in the times that we do waver.

Self-compassion is understanding the myriad reasons why you've behaved and chosen the way you have in the past, but it's also accepting that you will not be perfect moving forward. There is no amount of work and or mental effort that could bring us to a point where we will be forever sure we will always choose the best path and never again make a "mistake."

For a person with SUD, there may be times when they find themselves in the car on the way to the liquor store or to that one old acquaintance's home who still uses and always seems to have enough to share. They may be thinking of how simple and easy drinking or using would be and imagining that relief from their discomfort.

Even in these moments when relapse seems so close, your person can still make a U-turn. They can still choose recovery.

Many times, I've heard people share about instances of arriving at the liquor store parking lot—and then just sitting there, thinking about why they are there. The inner voice of "I just want a drink" can be loud, but with space and practice, it can also be reasoned with. They can say to themselves, "I don't actually want a drink. I just want relief from how uncomfortable I feel right now. This worked for that in the past, but I don't want to do that anymore, so what else can I do?"

That space of self-compassion gives them room to turn the car around.

The process of recovery that families go through will also have those same moments of wavering. There will be times when you slam a door, get caught off guard by a phone call, or are presented with a choice that doesn't fit within the action plan. We can say,

"You know what? I'm really working hard not to react like that, and I'm not proud of how I showed up yesterday."

We also can turn the car around. When we have learned that change is possible, it's a skill we don't lose, and we can still change and recover ourselves so we can show up better the next day and the next.

Every recovery journey is unique, and when it's your life you're trying to manage, there's no one-size-fits-all action plan. You wouldn't expect someone you love to be able to react in the best possible way to every possible curveball, so we can also have compassion for ourselves when we need more time to reflect and choose differently.

One family I worked with had a change of circumstances that didn't fit neatly in the stages of recovery. A young man in recovery from SUD with issues around both alcohol and opioids had sustained a serious and very painful injury. Nearly anyone leaving the hospital with this manner of injury would be given opioids as pain management, as the months ahead of physical recovery would continue to be extremely painful.

Of course, this is a very difficult choice for someone in SUD recovery and not one to be taken lightly. The young man discussed it with his family and made the case that he would need the medication to manage his pain. But during the discussion, one member shut down and wouldn't engage in the discussion. Going silent had been an old defense mechanism that felt like a holdover from previous issues. It's not how she would want to be present in that moment, but when he shared his reasoning, she froze. Everything he was saying, even in this different situation and circumstances, resonated with all his old drug-seeking and justifying behaviors. Of course it did—her reaction made sense because the parallel was there and the situation was complicated and precarious.

It wasn't black and white; there was no clear-cut correct way to respond. Her freezing and shutting down the conversation were not "mistakes," but she still needed to make a U-turn. The relationship couldn't be left in that silent, frozen place. We were able to talk together about how she could have been authentically curious and responded differently, and she was able to explore and reflect on how it had affected her and what type of partnership would help her be more supportive and less reactive.

After some time had passed, she was able to reconnect with him and ask if he was okay with going back to the conversation. She had some thoughts she wanted to share.

There will be times when you react with mechanisms that didn't serve you well in the past, whether it's shutting down, yelling, slamming doors, using guilt to try to control your person's behavior, or any number of reactionary responses to circumstances that don't really help address the problem. There will be steps back, but when you have learned how to make a U-turn, you can *always* do so. You can reflect, reassess, find your intention, and return to the situation with your tools to engage better.

My son worked for a time for a wilderness therapy organization, facilitating outdoor experiences for struggling adolescents and young adults in a therapeutic setting. It was intense work—out in the field for eight days at a time and home for six. Being in nature is a central passion in his life, so he absolutely loved it, but it came with many challenges.

While he loved the work, the culture around off-times and site trainings was not safe or inclusive for him, and yet they came with pressure to attend. In these events, most of the other staff would socially gather and consume casually and habitually. My son was in recovery and feeling secure in his recovery, but he did not want to be surrounded by that behavior in a captive environment where no one else was sober. He would generally do his own thing in these times, often with just one of the other guides. This garnered some criticism from his employers, who saw the gatherings as important to team building. Thankfully he was able to advocate for himself in this moment, explaining why that environment was not an emotionally safe place for him to spend time, especially regularly.

Even though this was a bit of a sour note in a job that he otherwise loved, it was also an opportunity to be a model for change for others. He demonstrated how reflection, growth, and change can look, and though his advocacy didn't bring about a total U-turn in the company culture, it moved the needle.

On one of his shifts over the winter season, he was also presented with a difficult opportunity to exercise self-compassion and appreciated his ability to make a U-turn in his life.

It was Christmas Eve, and an unexpected rainstorm had passed through the area of Utah where they had been camping. In the winter, camping in snow is to be expected, and the group was well equipped to stay warm, safe, and relatively comfortable in the snow. But rain was another story. The weather became a major hassle for the group as their plan for a peaceful time spent in nature quickly turned into a cold, wet nightmare.

My son took on the responsibility of getting all the sleeping bags clean and dry, which meant that he spent that Christmas Eve, alone, wrangling forty sopping-wet sleeping bags at a public laundromat. Deeply disappointed to be inside under fluorescent lights instead of doing what he loved outdoors, he felt terrible about the way he was spending his holiday. In short, it sucked, and he was feeling sorry for himself.

To make everything worse, a man came in, apparently unhoused and intoxicated, and made a beeline for the bathroom, clearly seeing the space as a place to use drugs. He thought of how what the man was doing would bring him relief from how he was feeling about his situation—how easy and simple a solution it would be to his discomfort. He then thought of those times in the past when he sought that kind of relief but found so much destruction. It was a familiar internal struggle: He wanted immediate relief despite understanding its potential harms. The brain never really forgets its old rationalizations, so those thoughts floated back up.

In the past, he had met those feelings and thoughts with judgment and self-criticism. He would tell himself that he sucked, and he couldn't believe the thought would even occur to him. This negative self-talk itself would spiral out. Every single time he returned to use or even thought about it, the judgment would start up again, worsening his discomfort and making it harder and harder to cope.

Blame and judgment aren't useful. They don't keep us safe, even from ourselves.

When things started to change for him and his recovery was making lasting progress, he didn't stop having thoughts about how using would be an easy way to take his discomfort away. The rationalizations weren't silenced. But instead of putting himself down with criticism, he began to meet these thoughts with compassion.

In that laundromat, he told himself, *Yeah, it makes sense that you would think about that. This sucks, and there were a lot of times that worked to make things suck less for a little while. But you don't have to do that. How else could you find relief?*

This is the simple power of self-compassion. It's not enough to just understand that a behavior can be harmful—if it were, none of this would be so hard. We also have to understand where the behavior comes from and forgive ourselves in order to strengthen our mindset and ultimately choose differently.

That work is what gives us the ability to make a U-turn.

Through self-compassion, my son could choose not to make his emotional state worse by berating himself or focusing solely on all the parts of his situation that were out of his control and infuriating. He could understand and forgive his cravings even as he was having them. He could reflect on what other ways he could self-soothe to get through the situation.

∿

When we begin a journey of self-reflection and awareness, it is natural that we will become more aware of decisions we wish we could go back and change. When we consider the "shadow sides" of our values—which are often the origins of those behaviors—they may feel at first like little cuts against our character. We can come to understand that our attempts to help were really attempts to control, that using words meant to shame others will never help them change, and that we can't make our well-being someone else's responsibility.

The patterns of our minds become deep in their repetition, like eroded ruts in our brains. It takes time and work to dig other paths for our thoughts and emotions. Hard circumstances will still come, and with that experience will come those same thoughts and emotions that led us astray before. Allowing room for compassion for yourself as those thoughts occur is exactly what gives you the strength to validate them, let them go, and choose a different action.

Throughout this book, I've outlined real and hypothetical examples of these behaviors, and you may have recognized parallels to things you or your family have experienced. This can be hard to relive, and it can be painful to look back at your past choices in a new light.

The goal of this reflection is not to look back on your past choices and rescore them with a harsher rubric. We are not trying to add new ways to consider yourself "wrong." This isn't about right and wrong or how to avoid the "mistakes" of the past.

Blame and judgment are not useful.

Rather, our shared goal is, with all the tools explored in this book working together, to learn a more sustainable and connected way forward. In this work, you can learn how to be more effective in meeting your intentions, having your intentions be heard and understood by both others and your full self, and celebrating loving connections with your people. This reflection on the past is about learning about yourself, exploring your motivations, and considering your choices more intentionally.

The way forward will not be snowplowed by this process. You will still face hard experiences and difficult choices. Understanding your intentions, limits, and needs may not guarantee that you know which choice will be successful. With every decision, you will not know how the chips will fall. Things will not come magically under your control, but with each experience, you can add more data to your understanding.

The choices may include what form of treatment to support, how you will engage and interact with your people, what boundaries you follow through with, how you respond if they return to use, and how you navigate your own recovery. They will be ongoing, and some of them may be less successful than you hope.

Every decision you make and experience you have is and will continue to be an opportunity to learn about yourself and the people in your life. Learning is acquiring more and more data and seeing how it fits into our greater understanding. This includes data about ourselves. We don't need to pass judgment on ourselves for what we chose before we had all the data by calling them "mistakes" or saying, "I screwed this all up" or "I failed." Through self-compassion and understanding our data, we can make different decisions that better align with what we want over the long term.

This data collection works for both you and your person with SUD.

Often, we hear people in various stages of recovery say, "Maybe I can just drink" or "Maybe I can just smoke weed." People who express this are feeling that they've regained a bit of self-control and seeing that there are others who at least seem to be able to use "in moderation." For my son and many others, each return to use provided more data that, no, they can't do that safely. For my son and many others who have experienced SUD, the data he collected showed him that his limit for safety and maintaining health and self-control was set at zero use. Others may have different lines, and collecting the data can show where they are.

That self-understanding allows for growth and change over time. Making a U-turn in your behavior doesn't have to be a complete rewrite of your daily life from one day to the next. Often, U-turns start small.

When a phone call or meeting doesn't go the way you wanted, you can model a U-turn by starting the next communication by acknowledging that you were reactive and didn't show up in a way that was helpful. You can share what it was about *you* that initiated your reaction. You may ask for space around that topic in the future. The first step is simply acknowledging that you've had some time to reflect on the way you were yesterday or last week and would like to try again a different way. Following up that acknowledgment with follow-through by making a genuine change—no matter how small—and sticking with it the best you can shows that change is possible. It shows that you're in this with your person, not against them.

Sometimes, the U-turn you take is to better protect your own space and peace by following through with boundaries and limits. When you've found yourself stuck in a cycle of resentment and reactionary responses, you can find *something*—your hamburger—to make a change around and stick with it.

When my sons were little, one of them said to me, "We know that when you say maybe, you actually mean yes."

It took me aback. Firstly, because you don't always expect a five-year-old to shine such a light on your behavior like that, but second, because I knew he was right. I just wasn't sure at the time how to do things differently. In my journey, my U-turns were often centered around learning to say no or yes with my full throat and not a maybe-that-means-yes.

These may seem like trivial changes in the grand scheme and in the face of staggering and dangerous problems, but they move the needle and make progress, which allows space for *more* progress. There will be setbacks and new U-turns you may need to take down the road. Life just has a way of presenting us with challenges and hard experiences.

There's no destination, but the road becomes less scary when you know you can change direction.

CONCLUSION

IN MY LITTLE corner of Colorado, we don't get very impressive sunsets. With the Rockies forming a wall to the west, the sun tends to just disappear in the evening, casting us in sudden shadow. The brilliant display of painted sky is all on the far side of the mountains, with just a few minutes of pink-tipped mountains before dark.

The sunrise is a different story.

For a long time, nights were hard for me. Fear and worry made restful sleep difficult and, at times, impossible. And there was nothing to do but fret and try to make dark hours pass, which always seemed to stretch out endlessly.

I often rise a little before dawn, just as the sky is lightening from deep navy to purple. Dogs are always excellent alarm clocks and make for a good excuse to get out and stretch your legs while the world remains mostly quiet and still. In darker times, walking the dog was my relief from the long and tortuous night. I always feel a bit more myself when I'm busy, so walking the dog was the beginning of the time when I could finally get out and start occupying myself.

Thankfully, my nights are easier and more restful these days, but I still start most days with this early morning walk. I've got my path plotted out perfectly, and on clear mornings, I turn one particular corner to face east into the rising sun.

It is glorious and never fails to fill my whole mind and heart with its beauty. The bright orange orb sits on the horizon and paints the whole sky in brilliant slashes of red, orange, and deep yellow. The light pushes back the dark across the sky, slowly revealing the beautiful light blue and the irregular shapes of the clouds. The warmth spreads amazingly quickly and caresses your face and hands.

Talk about awe.

There were times when that sunrise was a lifeline for me, an experience of beauty and peace that I desperately needed to feel each day. It meant I had made it through another night. It meant the glory of the world was still there, and I could still experience it. The gratitude I felt for those morning walks sustained me. It grounded me to remember that no matter how long the night seemed, the sun would rise.

Even now, the sunrise is something I don't miss if I can help it.

So much in this world is out of our control, everything from the tidal ebb and flow of day and night to the actions of everyone around us. It can make us feel helpless, but if we work at it, we can make room for awe, gratitude, and the strength to make the best choices that are available to us.

When presented with problems, we often reach for solutions that involve "fixing" what feels like the central issue. We look for how-tos and troubleshooting guides. The things our people do are among those things that are outside of our control, which is why this has not been a *How to Get Your Person into Treatment* manual. I would guess that in your search for practical advice on handling this difficult trial life has presented you with, you weren't expecting to read, "Make time for sunrises." That's completely understandable.

In a state of frantic need and fear, that advice may sound pretty thin. But in the journey of recovery, we can step *out* of that frenetic state. For you, it may not be sunrises or ruby-throated humming-birds. Perhaps it's the warm scent of rising bread, affection from a pet, or a perfectly timed joke. Making room for experiences that give you a sense of awe, peace, and joy is one part of the greater healing journey, whatever that may look like for you individually. It gives you both reason and energy to heal, independent of what we want from our people, especially when they are struggling to find that reason to heal for themselves.

As I said in the opening of these pages, the subjects explored in this book—reflection, psychoeducation, boundaries and agree-ments, ambiguous grief and tragic optimism, and self-compassion—are not steps but rather tools for you to use collectively as you work to make your life more sustainable, even through long nights where you feel helpless.

These tools are not the kind to be used to solve rarely occurring problems and then stored away in the bottom drawer. Rather, these tools can be carried with you wherever you go, and with them, you can adopt a new way to be, a new way to move forward. They can serve you through this healing path and help you face new chal-lenges as they come with resilience and strength. In the face of all the things we can't control, we can empower ourselves with one thing—the way we respond.

While we can't control others' actions and decisions, it is clear that we can be an influence, just like others have influenced us. Influence can be enormously powerful, but it is also delicate because it is, in a sense, a collaboration.

Control is an act of force, not love. Trying to bring about change through force will be met with resistance, rejection, or even counterattack. Force is not how we lead people to find themselves again but how we lose them.

Influence, on the other hand, is an invitation.

Think of those who have influenced you. You have seen models for ways of being that inspired you to improve. They didn't make you want to be better because they told you to be better. They lived it, and in seeing them experience that better way, you wanted it too.

You want your person to be better, but that is not enough. They have to step forward for themselves for that to work. To be a positive influence, we have to show what better looks like, what it looks like to be resilient, thoughtful, responsive, clear in our communication, kind in our words and actions, able to make deliberate changes in our patterns, and able to find peace. To influence our loved ones in that direction, we must first exemplify what that looks like.

We may be able to see that substance use is standing in their way. One thing that may be keeping them from that better way of being could very well be their substance use, but lifting that piece of their experience out of the whole won't bring about that better way of being all on its own. No part of our human experience happens in a vacuum, separate from all else.

In the families I work with, their person may not be ready to confront their use as something standing in their way. Others have started to contemplate that possibility but haven't yet been able to take real steps in that direction. Others have sought help but haven't managed to stay with the treatment.

Wherever your person is, connecting with them in a positive way can have an impact and influence them in a way that is much more foundational and essential than simply getting them a step closer to sobriety.

Moments of connection may be small, but their influence over time can be quite powerful.

Sharing thoughts on a recent movie, talking about positive hobbies, or even being together for a period of shared quiet time creates space for the connection to be felt and reinforced. That feeling of connection can build over time and become something your person will want more of—that you both will want more of.

This naturally invites your person to reflect on times when the connection does not come in that way. If they want more of that connection, they may have to make choices about how they are showing up for the relationship. That reflection is often the first step toward their healing.

That connection may be the reason they need to start their own work.

This is often not as easy as having tea or making time to chat over a card game. Their past behavior may have caused you genuine stress and pain, and your reactions in the moment may have created a back-and-forth history and pattern that can take a lot to break free from. Regardless of how it started, we all share the burden of making our connections to each other something worth showing up for. When we share the burden of change, we let go of the futility of trying to control the circumstances and open up possibilities for positive influence.

Creating these connections can require all of the tools discussed throughout this book, working in tandem.

To understand and feel empathy for them despite their behavior, we look to understand their psychology as much as we can. To understand our reactions and how we need to change, we acknowledge our grief and treat ourselves with compassion and patience. To disrupt painful patterns in our relationship, we work on our communication, our boundaries, our listening and understanding skills, and our capacity to acknowledge the patterns we're participating in may be part of a very long cycle.

All of these things working together have the united purpose of developing positive connections with our people and ourselves.

The main purpose is not to get our person to stop drinking or using, though that might be a secondary outcome. There is no 100 percent effective way to get someone to recover from their SUD, but we have found that the odds of long-lasting recovery are much, much higher when families engage in the process.

The connections we feel to each other are our reasons for

wanting better for each other and ourselves, and sharing that connection—and the burden of maintaining it—can generate the strength we all need for it to happen.

Older approaches to treatment, including philosophies based on "detach with love," show an 11 percent success rate for long-term recovery. When connection is treated as central to the treatment and recovery process through family engagement and Parallel Recovery, the success rate rises to 64 percent.

That shows that influence *does* have a measurable effect. As Johann Hari famously noted, the opposite of addiction is human connection. When people have connections with others, that gives us all reasons for wanting to be better.

It takes a great deal of strength to fight against the neurochemical patterns created by SUD and sustained resilience to form new patterns that will last. The connections we have to each other are what provide not only a good enough reason to go through the journey of recovery but also a force that empowers us to see it through.

From an objective position, the outcomes of SUD and recovery can and will look very different. Each of us is on a unique path, so our challenges will be different, and the ways we can give our influence and how much it can be accepted and felt will differ greatly. But with these tools, you can be in a better place than you are today, and your person will experience your love as much as they are able to.

In my work with many families affected by SUD in a variety of unique circumstances, the "outcomes" of the work cannot really be weighed against each other. They can only be weighed against how things were before the families engaged with the work. There is no guarantee of how much your circumstances will change, but that is also not where the value of this work lies. These strategies are not methods for building a certain set of circumstances around you. The value of the work is in itself. It gives you space to find peace, the strength to have a connection with your person where they are now, and the possibility of having a positive influence. That shift happens within you and can ripple out and improve the lives of those around you, including your loved ones who are struggling.

One family I work with is experiencing very dire circumstances. Their loved one has used heavily for a long time and suffers from other mental disorders that exacerbate the issue. The drug use has significantly affected his brain. Attempts to get him to engage with professional help have been unsuccessful. His condition is so severe that it is unlikely he will ever be "healed" in any measurable sense, no matter where that imaginary benchmark is placed. These facts are devastating to his loved ones, and there is no sugar-coating them. Their pain in these circumstances is enormous, and it has broken their hearts.

The work of recovery for themselves has helped them weather this pain, as heavy and immutable as it is. For them, the work of radical acceptance has especially been a lifeline in this dark time. They know that he is not and will never be able to accept the "answers" they may have to offer him to improve his situation. They have been able to love him through this time with radical acceptance, and in that practice, they have had a small handful of days in which they could connect with him. They loved him and knew that he could feel it in these precious times, as few as they were.

His state of mind and health is such that their ability to have influence over his choices is very limited. The only thing really left for them is to love him in a way he can feel so that he will not be wholly alone and unloved. Their story is painful, but how they have navigated it also carries that influence forward to other families, showing them that radical love is *always* possible.

Even in the direst of circumstances, where the hope for measurable change in the situation is not in view, this work has the ability to give us these very real moments of connection. Even in these worst possible cases, *that* is worth working for. After all, when we are grieving for those who are lost to us, what would we give for just a handful more days with them? To love them and to know that they feel it?

They will not be part of that 64 percent "success rate" in recovery for their loved one, but even in these difficult realities, honoring connection is beyond worth it.

Stories like this family's are hard to hear, but they are also part of the reason why I have dedicated my life to working with families who have been impacted by SUD. They are every bit as much of the reason why I do what I do as the families I work with who see their loved ones through treatment and into recovery. As tragic as their circumstances are, their experience of this reality is better for the work that they have done in their recovery.

The very best method that families have for guiding and supporting people out of SUD is through engaging in Parallel Recovery, honoring our connections with each other, and empowering them to do the work. What we've also learned is that even when this method doesn't "work" to bring about that outcome, it's still worth doing. It may not be our disorder, but our recovery from the impacts of SUD and other experiences is worth working through.

Wherever you are, I hope through reading this book, you can start to see the framework for building a more sustainable and healthier way to move through your life. You deserve to feel happiness and peace, and you can do the work to carve the space for that for yourself, regardless of what struggles and obstacles the people you love have created for themselves and in your relationship with them.

You can start small, finding things to be grateful for in the way they exist right now, today. You can make a plan for developing a support system for yourself while you start this work, reflecting on your values, your role in this situation as it is, and how you can start taking those important pauses in order to do better.

This process of Parallel Recovery that I'm inviting you to embark on is not easy. There will certainly be hard choices and challenges to your comfort. It is nothing less than a process of learning a new way of being. It will be worth it.

The sun will rise in the morning.

And it will be glorious.

ACKNOWLEDGMENTS

To Noah, for inspiring the heart of this work.

To Luke and Tom, for your unwavering support, steady encouragement, and the grace you gave me to bring this forward.

To Amanda and Emily, thank you for helping shape these pages with care, clarity, and belief in the message.

To the Page & Podium Press team, your guidance and partnership have meant the world.

To the families who have trusted me with their pain, resilience, and hope, you are this book's heartbeat.

To the professionals who've been steady companions in this work—those who lead with heart, offer both challenge and comfort, and never forget the families at the center—your presence has shaped more than you know.

And to everyone who has walked alongside me—seen or unseen —thank you for being part of the journey.

ABOUT THE AUTHOR

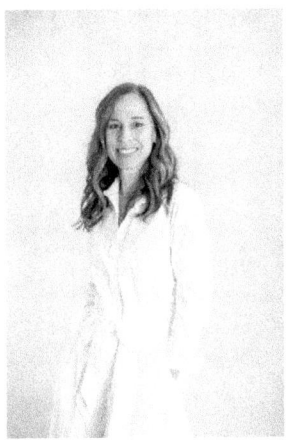

Lisa Katona Smith, MEd is the founder of Parallel Recovery-Family Recovery Services, and a nationally recognized advocate for families impacted by Substance Use Disorder (SUD). Drawing from her personal journey and over 20 years as a masters level educator, Lisa developed Parallel Recovery®, an innovative approach to fostering healing, sustainability, and connection. A TEDx speaker and trusted guide, she empowers families with compassionate tools to navigate recovery together. In Parallel Recovery, Lisa shares her transformative insights to help families thrive, one step at a time. She resides in Colorado with her family.

To learn more about Lisa and the work of Parallel Recovery, visit www.lisakatonasmith.com